Evidence-Based Clinical Practice in Nursing and Health Care

Assimilating research, experience and expertise

Alan Pearson
John Field
Zoe Jordan

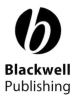

Blackwell
Publishing

Blackwell Publishing editorial offices:
Blackwell Publishing Ltd, 9600 Garsington Road, Oxford OX4 2DQ, UK
  Tel: +44 (0)1865 776868
Blackwell Publishing Inc., 350 Main Street, Malden, MA 02148-5020, USA
  Tel: +1 781 388 8250
Blackwell Publishing Asia Pty Ltd, 550 Swanston Street, Carlton, Victoria 3053, Australia
  Tel: +61 (0)3 8359 1011

First published 2007 by Blackwell Publishing Ltd

ISBN-10: 1-4051-5740-2
ISBN-13: 978-1-4051-5740-7

Library of Congress Cataloging-in-Publication Data
Pearson, Alan, SRN.
Evidence-based clinical practice in nursing and healthcare : assimilating research, experience, and
expertise / Alan Pearson, John Field, Zoe Jordan.
     p. ; cm.
Includes bibliographical references and index.
ISBN-13: 978-1-4051-5740-7 (pbk. : alk. paper)
ISBN-10: 1-4051-5740-2 (pbk. : alk. paper)
1. Evidence-based nursing.   2. Evidence-based medicine.   I. Field, John, RPN.   II. Jordan, Zoe.
III. Title. [DNLM: 1. Joanna Briggs Institute for Evidence Based Nursing and Midwifery.
2. Nursing Care–methods.   3. Evidence-Based Medicine–methods.   4. Models, Nursing. WY 100
P361e 2006]

RT42.P412 2006
610.73 – dc22
2006013659

A catalogue record for this title is available from the British Library

Set in 10/12.5 pt Palatino
by SNP Best-set Typesetter Ltd., Hong Kong
Printed and bound in Singapore
by COS Printers Pte Ltd

The publisher's policy is to use permanent paper from mills that operate a sustainable forestry
policy, and which has been manufactured from pulp processed using acid-free and elementary
chlorine-free practices. Furthermore, the publisher ensures that the text paper and cover board
used have met acceptable environmental accreditation standards.

For further information on Blackwell Publishing, visit our website:
www.blackwellpublishing.com

Contents

Preface   ix
About the authors   xi

1 The Evolution of Evidence-Based Practice   **1**
Introduction   1
Evidence-based health care (EBHC)   4
Evidence-based medicine   5
Evidence-based practice around the world   6
Evidence-based practice: beyond medicine   8
A multidisciplinary affair   9
The roles of consumers   10
Criticisms of the evidence-based approach   11
Conclusion   14

2 A Comprehensive Approach to Evidence-Based Health Care:
The JBI Model   **16**
Introduction   16
Health care evidence generation   18
Evidence synthesis   21
Evidence (knowledge) transfer   24
Evidence utilisation   25
Conclusion   25

3 What is Evidence for Practice?   **27**
Introduction   27
Feasibility, appropriateness, meaningfulness and effectiveness   28
Achieving a balance between evidence of effectiveness and other
    evidence interests for clinicians and consumers   30
The nature of evidence   31
Evidence for health professionals   32
Evidence for health consumers   34
Conclusion   35

4 Health Care Evidence Generation   **36**
Introduction   37
Guiding paradigms in research   38
The qualitative/quantitative debate   42
Paradigm, methodology and method   43
The quantitative research approach   43
The interpretive research approach   44
The critical research approach   45

Sources for evidence of feasibility   49
Sources for evidence of appropriateness   49
Sources for evidence of meaningfulness   50
Sources for evidence of effectiveness   50
Conclusion   50

5 Evidence Synthesis: The Systematic Review   **52**
Introduction   53
Overview of the systematic review process   54
The importance of systematic reviews of evidence   63
Finding the evidence   64
Study selection   69
Conclusion   70

**6 Evidence Synthesis: Critical Appraisal, Data Extraction and the
Synthesis of Findings**   **72**
Introduction   73
Critical appraisal of evidence   74
The limitations of critical appraisal   88
Data extraction   89
Data analysis and synthesis   92
Practical tools for systematic reviews   96
Conclusion   97

**7 Evidence Transfer: Writing Up a Systematic Review Report and
Developing Clinical Guidelines**   **99**
Introduction   100
The purpose of the systematic review report   101
Writing the report   102
What is a clinical guideline?   103
Medicine-specific guidelines   104
Nursing-specific clinical guidelines   104
Allied-health-specific guidelines   104
'Consensus' versus 'evidence'   105
Strategies for guideline development   105
The quality of the evidence   107
Grades of recommendation   108
Consumer involvement in guideline development   112
Guideline appraisal   113
The role of guidelines in practice   114
Practical tools for guideline development   115
Conclusion   116

8 Evidence Utilisation: Implementing Evidence-Based Guidelines   **118**
Introduction   119
Barriers to change   120

Changing practice   122
Evidence-based health care and practice change   124
The theory behind change   125
A process for change   125
Tools and strategies   127
Models for change   130
Knowledge translation   133
Evaluation   133
Conclusion   135

 9 **Evidence Utilisation: Clinical Audit**   **137**
Introduction   138
Clinical effectiveness   139
Clinical audit   139
Strategies to promote successful auditing   148
Writing an audit report   148
Practical tools for clinical audit   149
Clinical audit and research   151
Conclusion   152

10 **Evidence-Based Practice: Issues and Challenges**   **154**
Introduction   156
Evidence-based practice and the role of organisations   156
Legal and policy implications of evidence-based practice   158
Health care takes the lead . . . and others follow   162
Consumer participation   163
The rise and rise of information technology   164
Conclusion   166

References   168
Further Reading   172
Appendices   173
   Systematic Review Protocol Example   173
   Critical Appraisal Tools   177
   Data Extraction Tools   183
Index   187

Preface

Evidence-based health care (EBHC) is widely promoted internationally and is now a fundamental component of health planning, health services funding and the education of undergraduate and postgraduate health professionals in most countries. In medicine, nursing and the allied health professions, the Cochrane Collaboration approach to EBHC (focusing on evidence of effectiveness through the meta-analysis of randomised controlled trials) is well accepted. However, as useful as it is, this emphasis on evidence of effectiveness is recognised as a limitation by an increasing number of clinicians because it does not adequately take account of the broader interest of health-care professions in the human condition and human experience.

Most current texts on EBHC concentrate largely on effectiveness and on the 'Cochrane' approach to what constitutes usable evidence. There are, however, emerging alternatives and this book has as its organising framework the Joanna Briggs Institute Model of Evidence-Based Health Care. This model, developed by the Joanna Briggs Institute, recognises the three spheres of research, theory and practice as sources of evidence. Our aim was to develop a source book for students and practitioners of nursing and the other health professions that links evidence from diverse sources to the core of professional practice in health care: clinical decision-making and practice improvement.

Using the book

This book takes a practical approach to developing, implementing and evaluating practice based on 'evidence' in its broadest sense. It does this by describing the complexities of evidence-based practice without over-simplifying the issues and processes involved. Where necessary for a comprehensive understanding of the principles of evidence-based practice, the theoretical underpinnings are explained and explored. A number of devices are incorporated in the book for this purpose. For example, scenarios from practice are included to give the reader an opportunity to apply the principles and strategies examined in the book. As an adjunct to this process, a toolbox approach is incorporated in the various chapters to aid in the identification of the right tool for the particular task.

As well as examining the concept of clinical effectiveness and the Cochrane Collaboration approach to the meta-analysis of quantitative research findings, we consider other forms of evidence and describe how they can be used as legitimate sources of evidence for practice. The book also describes the development of condensed practice information sheets and clinical guidelines. It gives practical guidance on the implementation of evidence-based practice. Evaluation is also addressed, utilising the mechanism of the clinical audit.

The book has been written for those who are committed to basing their practice on the best available evidence. It gives practical guidance to students and practising health professionals on the processes involved in pursuing a broad, comprehensive approach to the identification, appraisal and implementation of evidence for clinical practice. Thus, the book will be of assistance to people involved in the delivery of health care at every level from student health professionals through senior clinicians to those charged with the responsibility for managing health-care services.

Chapter 1 describes the development of evidence-based health care internationally and Chapter 2 overviews the JBI Model of Evidence-Based Health Care. Chapters 3 to 9 examine the components and elements of the JBI Model of Evidence-Based Health Care (What is Evidence for Practice? Chapter 3; Evidence Generation, Chapter 4; Evidence Synthesis, Chapters 5 and 6; Evidence Transfer, Chapter 7; and Evidence Utilisation, Chapters 8 and 9). Chapter 10 considers the future of evidence-based practice.

Each chapter includes additional resources for those who wish to explore further particular aspects of evidence-based health care.

Alan Pearson
John Field
Zoe Jordan

About the Authors

Professor Alan Pearson *PhD FRCNA FAAG FRCN RN*

Professor Alan Pearson has extensive experience in nursing practice, nursing research and academic nursing. Professor Pearson has been an active researcher since 1981 and is known internationally for his pioneering work on the establishment and evaluation of nursing beds in Oxford, UK, from 1981–1986 and for his ongoing work, which emphasises the centrality of practice and evidence-based practice.

Professor Pearson was appointed to Australia's first Chair in Nursing at Deakin University in 1986; was Foundation Professor of Nursing at the University of New England from 1992–1995; was Foundation Professor of Clinical Nursing at The University of Adelaide from 1995–1999; and was appointed as a Chairperson of the Commonwealth Aged Care Complaints Resolution Committee in 1998.

He has conducted a large number of competitively funded research projects. As well as his ongoing research in the fields of aged care, nursing history, and brain death and organ donation, Professor Pearson was founder of the Joanna Briggs Institute. He is currently Executive Director of the Institute, and Professor of Nursing at The University of Adelaide. Professor Pearson is Editor of the *International Journal of Nursing Practice* and has authored over 40 books and over 120 journal articles. He is active in developing and promoting evidence-based practice at the state, national and international levels.

John Field *DNE (CumbCHS) BLegSt (Macq) GCertManag (NE) FRCNA FCN RN*

John Field is a nurse and a lawyer who has been involved in mental health nursing and academic nursing for more than 30 years. With qualifications in nursing, law, education and management, John is currently a Senior Lecturer at James Cook University in Queensland, Australia, where his teaching and research are focused on health law and ethics, evidence-based practice, and nursing education in developing communities. Since being appointed as a senior lecturer at the University of New England in 1991, he has held such posts as Head of School, Health Sciences, University of New England; Director, International and Flexible Learning Unit, The University of Adelaide; and Director, International Programs Unit, School of Nursing and Midwifery, La Trobe University. For much of the past decade his professional work has been focused on the development and administration of nursing education programmes in such countries as Bangladesh, Bhutan, Hong Kong, Singapore, and Sri Lanka.

Zoe Jordan *MA BA*

Zoe Jordan has been actively involved in the field of health research and communication for the last eight years. She has a Master of Arts (Communication Studies) for which much of her work was focused on utilisation of the mass media for the effective and accurate transfer of information. Having worked at the Joanna Briggs Institute for six years, Zoe has been intrinsically involved in the systematic review process, both as a reviewer and as a co-ordinator of the peer review process. She is currently the Manager, Communications and Consumers, at the Joanna Briggs Institute. This service endeavours to provide current, reliable, evidence-based health information to consumers of health care. Her work at the Institute focuses on contemporary approaches to health communication, specifically with regard to the emerging interrelationship and convergence of communication, media and culture in the context of a global society.

Chapter 1

The Evolution of Evidence-Based Practice

'Evidence-based medicine is the conscientious, explicit and judicious use of current best evidence in making decisions about the care of individual patients. The practice of evidence-based medicine means integrating individual clinical expertise with the best available external clinical evidence from systematic research. By individual clinical expertise we mean the proficiency and judgement that individual clinicians acquire through clinical experience and clinical practice.' – David Sackett

This chapter discusses:

- The purpose of evidence-based health care (the achievement of global health).
- The components of evidence-based health care (addressing the evidence, the preferences of the client, the context of care and the professional judgement of the practitioner.
- The development of evidence-based health care internationally.
- The pros and cons of evidence-based health care.

Introduction

Health professionals are often expected to work as part of a multidisciplinary team in order to provide appropriate care to their patients. This requires an extensive repertoire of skills. Two vitally important skills within this repertoire are first, the ability to examine the evidence related to a proposed course of treatment, and second, the ability to apply that evidence in their practice. As demonstrated in this chapter, this is not an easy task.

Throughout this text, you will be provided with scenarios regarding the management of a patient who is attempting to quit smoking. Smoking cessation is only one example of the many situations in which a multidisciplinary approach is necessary to effectively manage a condition (in this case, requiring input from disciplines including medicine, nursing, mental health, pharmacy and more). It is also an example where a comprehensive understanding of the importance of evidence-based practice will contribute to better patient outcomes. It has been chosen in order to provide a practical context in which to frame and demonstrate the theoretical concepts presented throughout this text.

In practice . . .

You are required to attend a female client called Lucy who is seven months pregnant. Lucy is a smoker and has come to the health service for a regular check-up. She is distressed, however, as she has read that smoking during pregnancy can lead to possible complications. She has read and understood information about quitting over the years but has still been unsuccessful in her attempts to stop.

Why is it that having evidence (knowledge) about health-promoting behaviours is so frequently insufficient to induce individuals to change their own behaviour to preserve or improve their health?

When detectives investigate a crime, they search for evidence to solve that crime. They need to locate evidence to identify a suspect; then they need further evidence to persuade the public prosecutor to charge the suspect with the alleged crime; then they need still more evidence to prove the guilt of the suspect to the court in order to obtain a conviction. This is not unlike the processes involved in practising evidence-based health care. Just as the detective searches for evidence to solve the crime, health care professionals look for evidence to guide them in their practice. Just as the detective must have evidence to establish the accused person's guilt, the health care professional must have evidence to support the proposed activity, intervention or course of treatment. This requires a rigorous and comprehensive search for information that will assist them to select and deliver the most effective or beneficial form of care to their clients.

In an information-rich age, copious amounts of research and information are available to health professionals on an ever-growing number of topics. Unfortunately, this wealth of information means that it can be a difficult and time-consuming process to appraise and synthesise all of the available research from which to extract the evidence upon which a decision may be based. Note that the value of research lies in the evidence that it provides. The environment in which health professionals practise is unpredictable, and having the ability to comprehend the language not only of the discipline but also of research is no small achievement. Comprehension is only half the battle, however, because it is also necessary for health professionals to possess the ability to access, appraise and implement this new knowledge as appropriate in clinical practice.

These skills are essential at every level of health care practice. Whether you are a newly qualified practitioner engaged in delivering hands-on care, or a senior manager in a health service organisation, you need to be aware of the current literature; you need to have the ability to evaluate the quality of the available research; and you need to have the ability to implement practice that is supported by research. The extent to which you can accomplish each of these professional responsibilities will vary depending upon such factors as your position in the organisation and your level of autonomy in practice, but the components of the process remain the same. The organisation will have in place procedure manuals and protocols that prescribe practice, and the processes for ensuring currency of practices in terms of available evidence will obviously have an impact on the capacity of the individual to implement practice change. Collaboration at all levels of the organisation is essential to optimise practice.

It is the challenges associated with assimilation of the avalanche of available information that we address throughout this book. We recognise that for many health professionals (as for many other disciplines) theory and practice can often seem worlds apart. In this book we endeavour to bring them closer together so that for practising health professionals, they are a seamless part of every day activity.

Professional practice and the use of evidence

Medical practitioners, nurses and allied health professionals are afforded a high status in most societies. They are seen to possess a specialised knowledge base; specific skills in delivering health care; a commitment to service to patients; and a commitment to 'being in touch' with new and emerging evidence about health, illness and ways of helping people to achieve optimal health.

Generally speaking, society expects health professionals to base their practice on the best available evidence – even if this expectation is not expressed in these specific words. Here in this chapter we examine the emergence of formalised evidence-based health care practice as an international movement and discuss the relationship between this movement and professional practice. Basing practice on evidence has been claimed to be a feature of modern health care – but the reality is that this claim has not always been reflected in everyday practice.

Many health care practitioners have based their practice on what they learned in medical, nursing or allied health schools; on trial and error in practice; or on reading single study reports in a small number of journals. None of these approaches to practice is appropriate in an age of rapidly changing knowledge. The material learned as an undergraduate student becomes outdated very quickly and the results of a single study, or of trial and error, do not stand up to the rigorous standards that are expected by society. Hence, the emergence of the evidence-based practice movement – a movement designed to capture and summarise the mass of available information, and to distil from that mass useable information to inform busy practitioners when they make clinical decisions.

Dawes et al. (1999) argue that the combination of clinical overload and information requirements inhibits health professionals from achieving practice that is evidence based. In recent years the demands on health professionals have increased dramatically to a point where the responsibilities of a clinician can now seem overwhelming. These increased demands have come from patients, from politically determined structural changes in the health care system, and from the rapid expansion of information related to health care practice. Busy health professionals are now hard pressed to find the time to complete everyday tasks, let alone evaluate and change practice, and yet the development of practice is central to their professional life. After all is said and done, the *raison d'être* for health care practice is improved outcomes for the consumers of health care.

It is for this reason that the evidence-based health care movement has captured the imagination of many health care practitioners who see its potential for achieving improved outcomes for consumers while easing the burden on practitioners by developing mechanisms for the expeditious distillation and dissemination of evidence as knowledge. In the remainder of this chapter we will briefly recount the history and development of the evidence-based health care movement around the globe.

In practice . . .

Lucy was unsuccessful in quitting smoking in spite of having evidence of its harmfulness and of effective strategies for cessation. What strategies could you employ both to assist Lucy to quit smoking and to ease her distress?

Learning activity

Think about your typical day in the clinical setting. Write a one-page plan for your day at work and include in it as much detail as possible. Include in this plan your decision-making processes, from the start of your day to the end. How might an evidence-based approach impact on any or all of the activities that occur during your day's work?

Evidence-based health care (EBHC)

Decision-making in health care has changed profoundly over the years for both health professionals and consumers. Not only are they expected to make decisions that are based on the best available evidence, but they are also required to review such decisions as new evidence comes to light. The promotion of evidence-based practice, which stems from A. L. Cochrane's work in relation to evidence-based medicine, is gaining momentum in most westernised countries. Cochrane drew attention to the lack of information about the effects of health care, with particular reference to medicine, and suggested that:

> 'It is surely a great criticism of our profession that we have not organised a critical summary, by specialty or sub-specialty, adapted periodically, of all relevant randomised controlled trials.' (Cochrane, 1979)

Cochrane argued that as resources for health care are limited, they should be used effectively to provide care that has been shown, in valid evaluations, to result in desirable outcomes. In particular, he emphasised the importance of randomised controlled trials in providing reliable information on the effectiveness of medical interventions.

The movement towards evidence-based health care practice thus focuses on the need for all health professionals to use those interventions that are supported by the most up-to-date evidence or knowledge available. The evidence-based approach acknowledges the difficulties faced by busy practitioners in keeping up to date with an ever growing literature in health care and emphasises the importance of providing them with condensed information gathered through the systematic review of the international literature on a given topic.

Although there is an international focus on a formalised and multidisciplinary approach to the conduct of systematic reviews and dissemination of evidence-based information, until recently most activity has been in relation to medicine, and evidence-based practice has largely been a synonym for evidence-based medicine. This is changing, however, with nurses and allied health professionals taking increasing interest in establishing an evidence base for their practice, and pursuing strategies to utilise evidence in practice.

Evidence-based medicine

The development of evidence-based medicine has been rapid since its emergence in the early 1990s and has primarily been led by Professor David Sackett of the University of Oxford. Evidence-based medicine (EBM) has been defined by Sackett and colleagues (1996) as:

> 'The conscientious, explicit, and judicious use of current best evidence in making decisions about the care of individual patients. The practice of evidence-based medicine means integrating individual clinical expertise with the best available external clinical evidence from systematic research.' (Sackett et al., 1996)

Sackett and Rosenberg (1995) argue for the need to base medical practice on the best possible evidence; to critically appraise research reports for validity and usefulness; and to incorporate the rapidly growing body of evidence into medical practice. They suggest that EBM is concerned with five linked ideas:

- That clinical and other health care decisions should be based on the best patient, population and laboratory-based evidence.
- The nature and source of the evidence to be sought depends on the particular clinical question.
- The identification of the best available evidence requires the application of epidemiological, economic and bio-statistical principles plus pathophysiology and personal experience.
- This identification and appraisal of the evidence must be acted upon.
- There should be continuous evaluation of performance.

This evidence-based approach to medicine draws on the activities of numerous specialist groups from across the world, linked together to form the Cochrane Collaboration.

The Cochrane Collaboration

The Cochrane Collaboration focuses on the systematic review of randomised controlled trials for specific medical conditions, client groups or specific health professional interventions. The collaboration links review groups internationally and offers training and support to such groups. Review groups commit to an ongoing process of systematic review in a specific area, and this involves:

- Determining the objectives and eligibility criteria for including trials.
- Identifying studies that are likely to meet the eligibility criteria.
- Tabulating the characteristics and assessing the methodological quality of each study identified.
- Excluding studies that do not meet the eligibility criteria.
- Compiling the most complete set of data feasible, involving the investigators if possible.
- Analysing the results of eligible studies, using a meta-analysis or statistical synthesis of data if appropriate and possible.
- Performing sensitivity analyses if appropriate and possible.
- Preparing a structured report of the review that states the aims of the review, describes the materials and methods used and reports the results.

Review groups also engage in a continuous process of updating reviews. Although the Cochrane Collaboration caters for other interests (including non-medical groups) such as certain categories of health service users, groups of health professionals, settings for health care, and classes of intervention, the involvement of nurses and allied health professionals has, until recently, been limited.

Evidence-based practice around the world

Developments in health care in most westernised countries over the past ten years have been driven by a desire to contain costs and to increase effectiveness. The introduction of the notion of 'best practice' relates closely to this focus on clinical and cost-effectiveness, and 'best practice' is being increasingly linked to the need to base practice on the best available evidence. In North America high-cost research and development programmes have been funded to develop clinical guidelines generated from systematic reviews and medical practitioners have been encouraged to utilise the condensed information within these guidelines in their daily practice. Until 1996 the National Institutes of Health operated from a well-established strategy to review international literature and conduct meta-analyses to generate clinical guidelines based on best available evidence. Since 1997 clinical guideline development has been largely the province of the professional medical associations or colleges.

In Britain, the government has directed all major health care provider agencies to develop research and development (R & D) strategies; to establish R & D units; and to promote practices based on best available evidence. At the same time, the British government has established a number of centres for evidence-based practice and these are supported by health research centres such as the King's Fund for health services development. The strategic development of evidence-based health care in the UK developed quickly, with observable benefits. Since the establishment of the Centre for Evidence-Based Medicine in Oxford, a linked network of centres for evidence-based practice is evolving across the UK, with each centre contributing from a specific perspective. There are centres for evidence-based child health in London, surgery in Manchester and pathology in Nottingham, and others are planned.

Initially the contribution to health of nursing and the other allied health professions was not recognised in this initiative, but this was redressed by the establishment of a centre for evidence-based nursing at the University of York, which is also the home of the NHS Centre for Reviews and Dissemination. In addition, a number of large-scale initiatives focusing on clinical effectiveness and clinical audit have evolved as multidisciplinary endeavours, and medicine, nursing and allied health professionals are all very much involved in their activities. All of these linked centres bring together focused activities from a range of perspectives to comprehensively contribute to the whole – that is, **evidence-based health care** rather than **evidence-based medicine**.

In Australia, the Australasian Cochrane Centre was established at Flinders Medical Centre, Adelaide (as a joint programme of Flinders University of South Australia and The University of Adelaide) in early 1994. Funded by the National Health and Medical Research Council, the Centre was directed by Professor Chris Silagy who made a major contribution to promoting evidence-based practice in Australia and New Zealand. In March 1999 the Centre relocated to form part of the Monash Institute of Health Services Research at Monash University in Melbourne, Victoria. The Centre continues to be funded by the Australian Commonwealth Department of Health and Ageing, and is supplemented by funding from the New Zealand Ministry of Health. The international Joanna Briggs Institute was also established in Australia. With headquarters in Adelaide, South Australia, the Joanna Briggs Institute has collaborating centres in most Australian states, New Zealand, Asia, Africa, Europe and North America. Given the central role of nursing and allied health in health care delivery, and that the role of nurses and allied health professionals in evidence-based health care has been largely neglected, the Joanna Briggs Institute focuses on the need for an evidence base for nursing and allied health and on assisting health consumers to make informed health decisions.

For all countries it is important to get the maximum value out of every dollar spent on health care. For developing countries, however, this is of critical importance. They are faced with the dual problem of having acutely limited funds together with what can often seem to be an overwhelming array of challenges to achieving good health care. This is compounded by a limited capacity to determine what will be the most effective deployment of the limited funds they have available. In most cases, the development of health care in developing countries has involved emulation of the practices of the developed world, and in the main, this has meant emulation of the western world. If we are to pass on our practices to countries with far more limited resources than ourselves, then ideally only those practices for which there is good evidence of effectiveness will be transferred.

There are many opportunities for developed countries to assist developing nations to determine which practices are supported by evidence. Moreover, there will be a need to evaluate the implementation of practices in new contexts to determine the level of effectiveness in those contexts. Organisations such as the Cochrane Collaboration and the Joanna Briggs Institute are ideal vehicles for assisting in this way because of their international structures.

Evidence-based practice: beyond medicine

The impact of the principles of evidence-based medicine has been remarkable and, while not prominent, a growing number of related disciplines have sought to take up the challenge. The transfer of these principles has not always occurred smoothly as other disciplines have differed in focus and research base. Thus, responses to attempts at implementation have been varied. Whether nursing, mental health, allied health or even human resources, each has faced its own challenges in recognising the evidence-based movement and applying it within the context of their professional activities.

The establishment of organisations such as the Joanna Briggs Institute arose from the recognition of a need for a collaborative approach both to the evaluation of evidence derived from a diverse range of sources, including experience, expertise and all forms of rigorous research, and to the translation, transfer and utilisation of the 'best available' evidence into health care practice. It is generally accepted that contemporary health care is characterised by high levels of variability in practice and a serious lack of research utilisation. The Joanna Briggs Institute works with researchers, clinicians and managers to identify those areas where health professionals most urgently require summarised evidence on which to base their practice. The Institute brings together a range of practice-oriented research activities to improve the effectiveness of nursing practice and health care outcomes by:

- Conducting systematic reviews and analyses of the research literature.
- Collaborating with expert researchers and clinicians to facilitate the development of practice information sheets based on the systematic review of research.
- Participating in the dissemination and implementation of best practice information sheets and evaluating their impact on health care practice.
- Designing, promoting and delivering short courses in evidence-based health care for clinicians, researchers, managers and teachers.
- Offering direct fees for service consultancies to health service provider agencies to develop customised evidence-based practice training and evidence-based clinical information.
- Initiating primary research when indicated by the findings of the systematic review.
- Contributing to cost-effective health care through the promotion of evidence-based health care practice.
- Planning and organising regular colloquia to promote knowledge sharing.

Promoting the use of evidence generated through systematic reviews and clinical guidelines

The practical application of rigorously reviewed evidence is promoted through the development and dissemination of practice guidelines in most developed health care systems. Clinical practice guidelines consist of statements to assist practitioner and patient decisions about appropriate health care for specific clinical circumstances. They are systematically developed on the basis of consensus within expert groups. An increasing number of well-constructed, practical and evidence-based guidelines are being developed, largely within the United States, the United Kingdom, Australia and New Zealand.

Practice or clinical guidelines outline practices that can be supported by evidence. The guidelines are drawn from systematic reviews that set out to assay existing research to identify those practices that are demonstrably effective. They aim to identify what is now frequently referred to as 'best practice'. It is important to keep in mind that guidelines are not a substitute for clinical judgement. Rather, insofar as they provide a synopsis of effective practice, they are an aid for clinicians. It is true that some commentators argue that such guidelines can be used to limit or to prescribe the use of specific interventions. However, this possibility is ameliorated by the fact that in most cases the evidence does not identify one single intervention as being universally superior. Neither will the evidence necessarily support the lowest cost interventions and this too lessens the likelihood of guidelines being abused in the manner suggested by these critics.

Although it is now well understood that effective health care delivery is dependent upon all members of the multidisciplinary clinical team, evidence-based health care practice remains focused on medical practice. Similarly, there are still very few practice guidelines for many areas of health care practice that fall within the domain of nursing and allied health.

> **In practice . . .**
>
> Thinking about Lucy's plight, do you think that the foregoing brief account of evidence-based practice affords any possibilities for assisting you to help Lucy? Consider, in particular, the emphasis on the decision-making process and the nature of the evidence base.

A multidisciplinary affair

The relationship between research evidence and clinical practice has been tenuous to say the least in many cases, and this is true not only of medicine but also of nursing, mental health, allied health and so on. It is apparent that, despite wide recognition among the disciplines regarding the benefit of the translation, transfer and utilisation of research evidence in clinical practice, its success throughout health care has been erratic and inconsistent.

While the emergence of evidence-based practice has come about through the development of evidence-based medicine, the pattern of its influence on other disciplines has been varied. Trinder and Reynolds (2000) have suggested that those disciplines closest to the epicentre of the evidence-based movement have adopted its principles most enthusiastically and the response of those at the edges is fragmented and unpredictable.

During the course of the last decade a number of evidence-based nursing initiatives have emerged that have echoed the developments of evidence-based medicine. The Joanna Briggs Institute has already been described. It is one example of these initiatives. To a certain extent, the philosophies underpinning the evidence-based nursing movement have inevitably mirrored those of medicine. However, while certain parallels are obvious, more recently its evolution has seen not only the generation of broader definitions of what constitutes evidence for practice, but also significant undertakings with regard to facilitation of formalised approaches to the appraisal and synthesis of that evidence for utilisation in clinical practice.

Similarly, the evidence-based movement has impacted significantly on evidence-based mental health, not only with mental health professionals taking up the cause, but with mental health consumers demanding an evidence base for the effectiveness of treatments and interventions. The development of evidence-based mental health, as with many of the health disciplines, has been a lengthy process. However, its aims are nevertheless congruent with those of medicine with regard to reducing unnecessary variation in clinical practice.

Evidence-based practice began with medicine and, as has been described, it spread to nursing. It did not stop there, though, as the allied health professions have also embraced evidence-based practice. The reasons for adoption of evidence-based practice in all of the health disciplines are essentially the same, and they have been articulated earlier in this chapter. For the allied health professions, the reasons and requirements are essentially the same, but as for all health professions, the mechanisms need to be tailored to suit the particular profession. For the allied health professions this is evident, for example, through the structure of the Joanna Briggs Institute but also through the establishment of centres such as The Centre for Allied Health Evidence at the University of South Australia and journals such as *The Internet Journal of Allied Health Sciences and Practice*.

The roles of consumers

The evidence-based movement has not only affected health professionals. It has also had an impact on consumers of health care in terms of their information requirements, and their involvement in health care information development and utilisation more generally. A shift towards shared decision-making and evidence-based health care has generally meant the demand for valid and reliable health information for consumers has significantly increased. In order to achieve successful development and dissemination of evidence-based health information for consumers, innovative and unique approaches are required.

Increasingly, health communication activities involve consumers. The scope and depth of information available to both health professionals and consumers is highly variable, pointing to the need for high-quality, reliable, evidence-based information. In order to ensure that the translation, transfer and utilisation of evidence-based information to consumers occurs, it seems appropriate that organisations that provide health professionals with such information should be ideally situated to develop consumer-oriented information. The potential benefits of consumer involvement in these processes include improved compliance, reduced litigation, lower costs and improved outcomes. As consumers become more engaged with health care generally, it is anticipated that they will play an important role in the utilisation of evidence-based health information.

Criticisms of the evidence-based approach

The development of evidence-based health care has not been lacking in controversy. Criticisms of the evidence-based movement have been both practical and conceptual, ranging from issues surrounding accessibility of information upon which to base practice to whether or not evidence-based practice has the capacity to incorporate other forms of knowledge. Given that it is relatively easy to find papers adovocating the benefits of evidence-based practice, it is important here to focus on those that provide constructive criticism. Note the emphasis on 'constructive' criticism. This is because much of the criticism that EBP has evoked cannot be categorised as such. So, just what are the major criticisms of EBP?

(1) Health professionals are already doing it

There is a good deal of truth in this. Many health professionals do engage in evidence-based practice to the extent that this is possible given the constraints of time and the availability of quality evidence. However, there is substantial and compelling evidence against the existence of widespread evidence-based health care practice. First, in all health care sectors there are widespread and extensive variations in practice. This indicates that the one best way of doing something (if there is one best way) has yet to be determined for many of the services health professionals provide.

(2) Evidence-based health care is 'cookbook' health care

Evidence-based practice is concerned to coalesce the individual health professional's clinical expertise with the best available evidence in order to produce the best possible outcome for the particular patient. This necessarily involves taking into account the circumstances of the recipient of care. For example, although the evidence strongly suggests that tap water is as effective as more expensive cleansing lotions in cleaning wounds, the research from which this evidence has been derived was conducted largely in developed countries and should be treated with caution in developing countries where water supplies may not have been subjected to purification processes. Similarly, when a client strongly believes that the transfusion of blood from one person to another is wrong, her or his preference to not receive a blood transfusion may overrule the evidence that shows such a treatment to be the most effective.

Thus, genuinely evidence-based practise is ideally a client-centred approach which, when properly practised, is highly individualised. Critics contend that it has the potential (if not properly applied) to give rise to 'cookbook' care. The same pressures that produced the impetus for evidence-based health care in the first place could be responsible for mechanisms of evidence-based practice – such as clinical guidelines being used simply as a recipe for health care delivered without due consideration of the individual patient. However, we would argue that any practice that fails to take account of the individual patient is not evidence-based practice.

(3) Evidence-based practice relies on randomised clinical trials (RCTs) and meta-analyses

This is a valid criticism of the current style of evidence-based health care, with its emphasis on the results of randomised controlled trials and quantitative research, and its rejection of other forms of evidence. At the heart of the issue lies the critique of traditional science and the emergence of new paradigms for knowledge. Although its proponents would argue that evidence-based health care is not limited to these forms of traditional research, there has been considerable emphasis on RCTs and meta-analyses. This has drawn criticism from those health professions that regard qualitative research methods as equally valid forms of research. It is, of course, stating the obvious to note that nursing has been one of the more prominent advocates of qualitative research. Much of the research that has been done in and on nursing has been qualitative in nature.

A key tool of the evidence-based practice movement is the systematic review of research. However, qualitative research fares rather poorly in systematic reviews.

The question here becomes one of what is acceptable research in terms of generating knowledge that amounts to evidence for the purpose of informing practice. There are different answers to this question that reflect competing views on the subject. These views generally align with the various positions that characterise the longstanding debate between qualitative and quantitative researchers. This is clearly not an easily resolved argument, but it is vitally important in terms of ascertaining the value of research-generated 'evidence' to the practice of health care.

(4) There is no evidence

For largely historical reasons, the criticism that there is no evidence is even more applicable to nursing and allied health than to medicine. The gist of the complaint is that if we wish to engage in evidence-based practice, then there needs to be a body of research to provide the evidence on which to base that practice. However, in the great majority of systematic reviews that have been conducted on nursing and allied health questions, the result has been that the research is either non-existent or inconclusive. That is to say, there is no evidence one way or the other. For example, in a systematic review of research on the effectiveness of support for carers of people with Alzheimer's type dementia, the main result was that the research was inconclusive. The authors said that with '. . . the limited nature of the research evidence in mind, it is not possible to recommend either wholesale investment in caregiver support programmes or withdrawal of the same . . .' (Thompson and Thompson, 1998).

While the lack of evidence could be perceived as a barrier to evidence-based practice, it should be recognised that the need to base practice on evidence has only relatively recently become a concern for the health professions. Thus, identifying the lack of evidence is an important first step in developing the evidence base.

(5) Theory is more important than evidence in guiding practice

Flowing from the previous criticism is the argument that it is much more important that practice be well grounded in theory than in research. One of the main reasons for this is the rapidity with which 'evidence' – and especially technical evidence – becomes obsolete. It is not disputed here that practice should be grounded in theory. Nor would we contest the increasingly short lifespan for currency of evidence, and especially technical evidence. However, while practice should always reflect theory, it must be predicated on the best available evidence if it is to achieve optimal outcomes, which are after all the objective of practice. Evidence-based practice acknowledges that evidence is only 'the best available evidence' until it is supplanted by better evidence. Evidence-based practice addresses this by putting in place mechanisms for ensuring currency. Recurrent systematic reviews are one such method because such reviews not only capture the evidence of contemporary research but point to the gaps in the available evidence, thus identifying topics for further research.

These are the five principal criticisms of evidence-based practice. That there is critique and debate around this relatively new phenomenon is in itself healthy and to be encouraged. However, it is very early days for the evidence-based prac-tice movement as a whole, and it is especially early for nursing. There are very few easy answers with respect to the contentious issues associated with evi-dence-based nursing and in many cases the jury is likely to be out for some time to come. At this stage in its development, an open mind is fundamental to an objective appraisal. As you become more familiar with the nature and applica-tions of evidence-based practice your views will begin to crystallise, but at every point you will need to test them against the arguments of both the proponents and the critics. It is time now to begin a closer examination of evidence-based practice.

In practice . . .

Given the widespread activity associated with the evidence-based health care movement, it seems safe to assume that few practising health professionals could have
escaped at least some exposure to it. In your experience, are the above mentioned
criticisms of evidence practice valid? Have the proponents of evidence-based health
care done enough to either remedy or rebut these criticisms?

Conclusion

Rarely has a concept fired the collective imagination of health care professionals
and simultaneously sparked debate in the way that the notion of evidence-based
practice has, first for medicine and more recently for nursing and allied health.
Evidence-based practice is now a dominant feature of health care policy at all
levels. Simply defined, it is the melding of individual clinical judgement and
expertise with the best available external evidence to generate the kind of practice that is most likely to lead to a positive outcome for a client or patient. While
evidence-based practice is simple to define, there is nothing simple about the
process. The complexities of finding, appraising, summarising and utilising evidence are considered in the chapters that follow.

In practice . . .

Whether you are a student or a health professional, there will be aspects of this text
that may, at first glance, seem quite esoteric and remote from the actual daily delivery of care to consumers. However, a few moments' consideration should be sufficient for you to relate these concepts to practice, for much of the text is readily
identifiable. At the beginning of this chapter we introduced you to Lucy, and you
were confronted with her inability to quit smoking. Having regard for what you have
now learned about evidence-based health care, how might you respond to Lucy and
her dilemma? What are the steps you might take to ensure that she had adequate,
evidence-based information regarding smoking cessation?
   Now think about the key components of the emerging evidence-based movement
and consider whether any or all of these components have influenced practice in your
clinical field. What is the current relationship between the international evidence-
based movement and your field of professional practice?

Further reading and resources

If you would like to read further about evidence-based health care you might like to try
the following titles:

Dawes, M., Davies, P., Gray, A., Mant, J., Seers, K. and Snowball, R. (1999) *Evidence-Based
   Practice: A Primer for Health Care Professionals.* London, Churchill Livingstone Press.
Gupta, M. (2003) A critical appraisal of evidence-based medicine: some ethical consider-
   ations. *Journal of Evaluation in Clinical Practice* **9** (2): 111–21.

Muir-Gray, J.A. (2001) *Evidence-Based Health Care: How to Make Health Policy and Management Decisions.* London, Churchill Livingstone Press.

Sacket, D.L., Rosenberg, W., Gray, J.A., Haynes, R.B. and Richardson, W.S. (1996) Evidence-based medicine: what it is and what it isn't. *British Medical Journal* **312**: 71–2.

If you would like further information about some of the key organisations involved in the evidence-based movement, the following web sites may be of interest to you:

Agency for Health Quality and Research: www.ahcpr.gov/clinic/
King's Fund: www.kingsfund.org.uk/
Centre for Evidence-based Medicine: www.cebm.net/
Centre for Reviews and Dissemination: www.york.ac.uk/inst/crd/
Cochrane Collaboration: www.cochrane.org/index0.htm

If you would like more information about some of the organisations working towards the development and dissemination of consumer-related health information and participation, the following websites may be of interest to you:

Better Health Channel: www.betterhealth.vic.gov.au
Consumers Health Forum: www.chf.org.au/our_chf/index.asp
Health Matters: www.abc.net.au/health
Just Be Involved: www.joannabriggs.edu.au/consumer/index.php

Chapter 2

A Comprehensive Approach to Evidence-Based Health Care: The JBI Model of Evidence-Based Health Care

'I still believe in the possibility of a model of reality – that is to say, of a theory, which represents things themselves and not merely the probability of their occurrence.' – *Albert Einstein, 1951*

This chapter discusses:

* The Joanna Briggs Institute Model of Evidence-Based Health Care in relation to the identification, appraisal and synthesis of the best available research evidence to inform and improve global health.

Introduction

Although evidence-based practice in health care has a very short history relative to the length of time that health professions such as medicine and nursing have existed, it has been around long enough for it to become widely accepted. In the few decades since A. L. Cochrane coined the term 'evidence-based medicine' (EBM), the notion of grounding health care practice on the best available evidence has become embedded in the health care professions. That is not to say that it isn't controversial. It is, and the debates are considered in this text. While it is difficult to argue that health care practice should not be based on evidence, the debates are primarily around the methods and approaches of the evidence-based movement. In particular there is argument around what constitutes evidence. Reflecting its origins, EBM has restricted evidence to the outcomes of randomised controlled trials (RCTs), and this has been problematic for those professions that are interested in the human condition and in people's experience. Increasingly, however, this includes medical practitioners and this has opened the door to broader interpretations.

The limitation of the RCT-based approach became glaringly obvious when nursing attempted to adopt the EBM model. For nursing, the biomedical science is important but it is not the whole story. Biomedical knowledge alone is inadequate for the practice of nursing. A holistic approach necessitates acknowledgement of all aspects of the person. It involves understanding the experiences of individuals as well as having knowledge of diseases, pharmacology, and so forth. These areas lie beyond the scope of RCTs but it is possible to generate evidence through other methods. Much of the argument is about the quality of evidence generated through those other methods.

It was the need for evidence for nursing practice that was the genesis for the Joanna Briggs Institute (JBI). Since 1996 the Institute has been assembling that evidence. It has also been developing techniques for making sense of the evidence and for making it readily accessible to practitioners. Demand from other health professions saw JBI's activities extend beyond nursing to midwifery and the allied health professions. The JBI model that forms the organising framework for this book draws on all the knowledge and experience of JBI's first ten years.

In this book we examine the process of evidence-based practice as a form of clinical decision-making and we do so from a comprehensive perspective based on the JBI Model of Evidence-Based Health Care (Pearson et al., 2005). The JBI model describes the four major components of the evidence-based health care process as:

(1) Health care evidence generation
(2) Evidence synthesis
(3) Evidence/knowledge transfer
(4) Evidence utilisation

Each of these components incorporates a number of essential elements (Figure 2.1).

Evidence-based health care can be represented much as the dial of a clock – it is a cyclical process that begins with clinical questions, concerns or interests of clinicians or patients/consumers and then proceeds to address these questions by generating knowledge and evidence to effectively and appropriately meet these needs in ways that are feasible and meaningful to specific populations, cultures and settings. This evidence is then appraised and synthesised, and transferred to service-delivery settings and health professionals who then utilise it and evaluate its impact on health outcomes, health systems and professional practice.

In this introductory section each of the elements of the model is briefly explained and contextualised. Having surveyed the model as a whole, the book sequentially addresses in its remaining chapters the specific sections as we work around the clock. Eventually we will come to the end of time!

Evidence-based practice is essentially a form of clinical decision-making that focuses on achieving global health through applying the best available evidence. The achievement of improved global health is seen as both the goal (or endpoint) and the 'driving force' of evidence-based health care (Figure 2.2).

Evidence-based clinical practice takes into account the context within which care takes place; the preferences of the client; and the clinical judgement of the health professional, as well as the best available evidence (Figure 2.3)

That means that every health professional from every discipline, and at every level from novice to senior management, has a vested interest in this book. The nature of that interest will vary depending on the role of the individual, but the importance of clinical decision-making is fundamental to all levels of service delivery. The past decade has seen an avalanche of literature on the subject of

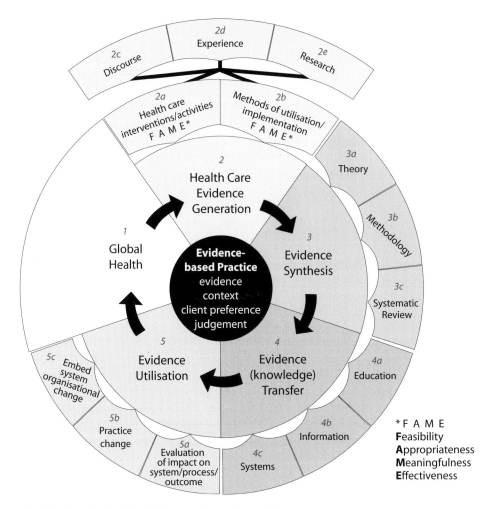

Fig. 2.1 The JBI Model of Evidence-Based Health Care.

evidence-based health care practice. This book does not merely offer a framework for understanding what evidence-based health care practice (EBHC) is, but for the practitioner it provides a clear account of how to apply it in practice. For the manager, it highlights the implications for attaining EBHC at an organisational level, including mechanisms for achieving the shift to an EBHC culture.

Health care evidence generation

Within the JBI Model of Evidence-Based Health Care, the generation of evidence enjoys its position at the top of the clock because it is first in time in the cycle of achieving evidence-based practice. To state the obvious, without evidence it

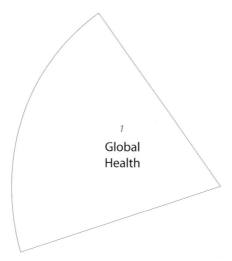

Fig. 2.2 Global health.

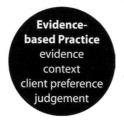

Fig. 2.3 Evidence-based practice.

would not be possible to have evidence-based practice. It is also at the top of the clock because of its singular importance to the process. Given the fundamental place of evidence in this form of clinical decision-making, it is essential that we clearly delineate what it is that we mean by evidence.

Evidence is not a simple concept, but in the JBI Model, and throughout this book, the term evidence will be used to mean the basis of belief; the substantiation or confirmation that is needed in order for us to believe that something is true (Miller and Fredericks, 2003). Health professionals seek evidence to substantiate the worth of a very wide range of activities and interventions, and thus the type of evidence needed depends on the nature of the activity and its purpose. The four types of evidence addressed in the JBI Model are merely introduced at this point. They are explored more fully in later chapters.

Evidence of 'feasibility'

Feasibility is the extent to which an activity is practical and practicable. Clinical feasibility is about whether or not an activity or intervention is physically, culturally or financially practical or possible within a given context.

Evidence of 'appropriateness'

Appropriateness is the extent to which an intervention or activity fits with or is apt in a situation. Clinical appropriateness is about how an activity or intervention relates to the context in which care is given.

Evidence of 'meaningfulness'

Meaningfulness is the extent to which an intervention or activity is positively experienced by the patient. Meaningfulness relates to the personal experience, opinions, values, thoughts, beliefs and interpretations of patients or clients.

Evidence of 'effectiveness'

Effectiveness is the extent to which an intervention, when used appropriately, achieves the intended effect. Clinical effectiveness is about the relationship between an intervention and clinical or health outcomes.

The evidence generation component of the model (Figure 2.4) identifies discourse (opinion), experience and research as legitimate sources for evidence or knowledge generation.

The sources of evidence are linked to the purpose of generation in evidence-based health care. That is to say, evidence will be generated to establish the feasibility, appropriateness, meaningfulness or effectiveness of a particular intervention, activity or phenomenon, and how this evidence is derived will have implications for how it can be utilised to change practice. Any indication that a

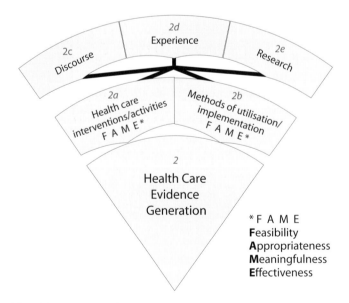

Fig. 2.4 Health evidence generation.

practice is effective, appropriate, meaningful or feasible – whether derived from experience or expertise or inference or deduction or the results of rigorous inquiry – is regarded as a form of evidence in the model.

Although any indication of effectiveness, appropriateness, meaningfulness or feasibility will be regarded as evidence, not all evidence will be given equal weight. The results of well-designed research studies grounded in any methodological position are obviously seen to be more credible as evidence than anecdotes or personal opinion; however, when no research evidence exists, expert opinion is seen to represent the 'best available' evidence. This is a clear departure from the model developed by the Cochrane Collaboration wherein evidence other than that generated through randomised controlled trials is disregarded.

Once evidence is generated, there is a need to ascertain what contribution the new evidence makes to the overall body of evidence relating to the intervention, activity or phenomenon. That is the focus of the second component of the JBI Model, that of evidence synthesis.

Evidence synthesis

Evidence synthesis is the evaluation or analysis of research evidence and opinion on a specific topic to aid in decision-making in health care. Put another way, evidence synthesis involves the pooling of results of research findings in such a way as to effectively determine just what interventions, activities or phenomena it is that the evidence supports. The process of evidence synthesis consists of three elements in the JBI Model: theory, methodology and the systematic review of evidence (Figure 2.5).

Perhaps because of its longer history, the science of evidence synthesis has developed most rapidly in relation to the meta-analysis of numerical data linked

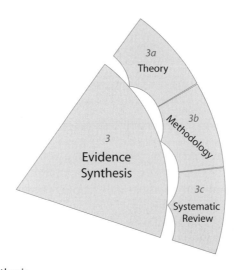

Fig. 2.5 Evidence synthesis.

to theories of cause and effect. Meta-analysis uses various statistical methods to combine the results of multiple different studies to produce a stronger conclusion than can be derived from any one of the studies on its own. The further development of theoretical understandings and propositions of the nature of evidence – together with the role of evidence in health care delivery and in the facilitation of improved global health – forms an important element of evidence synthesis in the JBI Model. For similar reasons, the increasing, ongoing interest and theoretical work on methods of synthesising evidence from diverse sources is an element of evidence synthesis in the JBI Model and one that is considered to be of central importance.

The third element of evidence synthesis is the operationalisation of methods of synthesis through the systematic review process. This element in the model is grounded in the view that evidence of feasibility, appropriateness, meaningfulness, effectiveness and economics are legitimate foci for the systematic review process; and that diverse forms of evidence (from experience, opinion, and research that involves numerical and/or textual data) can be appraised, extracted and synthesised (Pearson, 2004).

The systematic review and the synthesis of findings have their origins in quantitative psychology and the classical randomized controlled trial approach to clinical research in the health science fields. The JBI Model of Evidence-Based Health Care adopts a pluralistic approach to the notion of evidence wherein the findings of qualitative research studies are regarded as rigorously generated evidence and other texts derived from opinion, experience and expertise are acknowledged as forms of evidence when the results of research are unavailable.

The core of evidence synthesis is the systematic review of the literature on a particular condition, intervention or issue. The systematic review is essentially an analysis of all of the available literature (that is, evidence) and a judgement of the effectiveness or otherwise of a practice, involving a series of complex steps.

Systematic reviews occupy the highest position in current hierarchies of evidence because they systematically search, identify, and summarize the available evidence that answers a focused clinical question with particular attention to the methodological quality of studies or the credibility of opinion and text. The pluralistic approach of the JBI Model to evidence synthesis is inclusive of evidence that arises out of quantitative research, qualitative research, opinion and economic analyses.

The synthesis of the results of quantitative research

Statistical analysis (meta-analysis) may or may not be used in synthesising numerical data, and this depends on the nature and quality of studies included in the review. Meta-analyses of numerical findings provide precise estimates of an association or a treatment effect in reviews of effectiveness through the statistical synthesis of multiple studies. Key outcomes of the meta-analysis are the measure of effect, the confidence interval and the degree of heterogeneity of the studies synthesised.

The synthesis of the results of qualitative research

The term 'meta-synthesis' refers to a 'higher form of synthesis' or, as Light and Pillemer (1984) refer to it, the 'science of summing up'. Meta-synthesis is a process of combining the findings of individual qualitative studies (that is, cases) to create summary statements that authentically describe the meaning of these themes.

The synthesis of evidence arising out of expert opinion and text

Although the proponents of evidence-based health care would argue that the results of high-quality research are the only source of evidence for practice, this has drawn considerable criticism from clinicians. Clinicians argue that the nature of everyday practice demands an eclectic, pragmatic approach to conceptualising evidence. The 'consumers' of systematic reviews – those who practice within the health system – regard the opinion of experts and the views of experienced clinicians and their professional bodies as valid forms of evidence for practice. This is so particularly when some intervention or activity is required in practice, even though no evidence from research exists to indicate what, if any, intervention or activity will be most effective. The process seeks to locate the major conclusions in text that represent credible opinion.

The synthesis of evidence arising out of economic analyses

The synthesis of economic analyses or evaluations is a developing science. The lack of standardisation of systematic review methods is incongruous with the obvious need for these methods and the availability of existing effectiveness review methods that may be adapted in terms of searching, critical appraisal and data extraction (Carande-Kulis et al., 2000). Because of the paucity of high-quality studies and established methods to statistically synthesise studies, meta-analysis is currently not widely used to synthesise economic findings. However, it is still clearly useful to extract data from high-quality studies and present a summation of the results in a way that informs practice. Syntheses of economic evidence can provide important information for health care decision makers and there is ongoing work that identifies '. . . the promise, difficulties, and current limitations of the use of economic analyses by health care decision makers' (Pignone et al., 2005).

Having managed to synthesise the evidence, the question arises as to what is to be done with it. Now the clock ticks around to the next component, and we look at the vexed question of how evidence (knowledge) can be transferred to health care practitioners. It is these people who must ultimately determine whether particular evidence finds its way into practice, so it is essential that mechanisms are put in place to ensure the efficient dissemination of evidence as it becomes available.

Evidence (knowledge) transfer

This component of the model relates to the act of transferring knowledge to individual health professionals, health facilities and health systems globally by means of journals, other publications, electronic media, education and training, and decision support systems. Evidence transfer is considered to involve more than the dissemination or distribution of information. It is taken to include the careful development of strategies that identify target audiences – such as clinicians, managers, policy makers, consumers etc – and the design and implementation of methods to package and transfer information that is comprehensible and useable in decision-making. Fundamental to this process are:

- Developing understandable and actionable messages.
- Accommodating the context of a target audience's information needs.
- Delivering messages in cost-effective ways (including information technology, print material, meetings, workshops and training programmes).

The model therefore represents the evidence/knowledge transfer component as having three major elements, these being education and training, information delivery, and the transfer of evidence though organisational and team systems (Figure 2.6).

The transfer of evidence to those who are in a position to implement that knowledge in practice is obviously central to the EBHC process. This is so because it is the possession of that evidence or knowledge that enables health care practitioners to apply it in practice. It is the implementation in practice that is the focus of the next component of the JBI Model of Evidence-Based Health Care. In the model, this component is referred to as evidence utilisation.

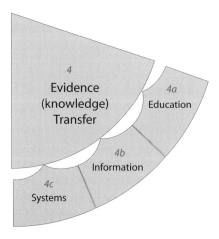

Fig. 2.6 Evidence/knowledge transfer.

Evidence utilisation

Since the objective of EBHC is optimal health care outcomes, it seems self-evident that the utilisation of best evidence for practice in practice will be the key to its success. It is this aspect of the EBHC process that is the concern of the component of the model termed 'evidence utilisation'. It relates to the implementation of evidence in practice, as is evidenced by practice and/or system change. Figure 2.7 identifies three elements of this component:

- Practice change.
- Embedding evidence through system/organisational change.
- Evaluating the impact of the utilisation of evidence on the health system, the process of care and health outcomes.

Evidence utilisation is highly influenced by factors such as available resources, provider education/expertise, and patient preference as well as available research (Dicenso and Cullum, 1998). When the evidence suggests the use of a particular intervention and clinicians wish to implement such an intervention, to do so requires organisational planning and decision-making processes. Organisational factors, in addition to individual clinician factors, contribute to these problems; staffing levels and mix, the availability of consultation services, and policies are all examples of factors beyond the individual clinician's control (Nicklin and McVeety, 2002). Grimshaw et al (2001), in a review of professional educational and quality assurance interventions, report that multi-faceted interventions targeting different barriers to change are more likely to be effective than single interventions.

Conclusion

Evidence-based health care is gaining acceptance globally. It is complex, sometimes misunderstood and frequently maligned. However, it will be evident from

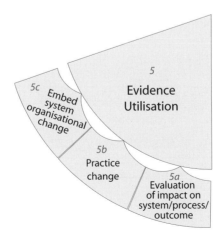

Fig. 2.7 Evidence utilisation.

the content of this introductory chapter that evidence-based practice involves giving consideration to the best available evidence, the context in which the care is delivered, client preference and the professional judgement of the health professional. Promoting and facilitating evidence-based health care, the JBI Model of Evidence-Based Health Care seeks to describe and critique evidence-based health care and its role in improving global health, within a logical conceptual framework. It represents EBHC as consisting of four major components of the evidence-based health care process:

- Health care evidence generation;
- Evidence synthesis;
- Evidence/knowledge transfer
- Evidence utilisation.

These components have been introduced in this chapter and they will be dealt with in detail in the various chapters of the book.

By this stage it will be apparent that what we are seeking to do in this book is to present a comprehensible model of evidence-based health care that takes account of its complexities, acknowledges the criticisms, and affords an understanding of the applications of evidence-based practice at all levels of health care practice. We have also sought to provide sufficient practical and theoretical knowledge to equip health care practitioners to engage in the process of evidence-based practice whatever their level of need, whether they be newly graduated practitioners, experienced clinicians or managers of health services. Readers may wish to simply dip their toes in the water of practice change, or they may wish to involve themselves in the wholesale development of an evidence-based practice culture in their organisation. At either extreme, or anywhere between, there is sufficient practical and theoretical assistance to equip the reader for the task.

Chapter 3

What is Evidence for Practice?

'*The most savage controversies are about matters as to which there is no good evidence either way.' – Bertrand Russell*

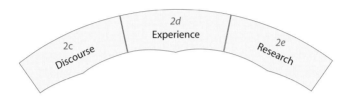

This chapter discusses:

- The evidence interests of practitioners (evidence of feasibility, appropriateness, meaningfulness and effectiveness).
- The sources of evidence used by health professionals.

In practice . . .

Joshua is a client who suffers from schizophrenia. He smokes very little when he is medicated and feeling well, but he is not always good at remembering to take his medication and it is then that he resumes smoking quite heavily. You are aware that research exists on different strategies to help individuals to quit smoking and feel that an individualised approach is necessary for this patient. Not only do you need to find information on effective strategies for smoking cessation, but you also need to find information that will account for the treatment's feasibility, appropriateness and meaningfulness in order to help Joshua.

As you read through this chapter, keep in mind Joshua's situation. At various points you will be asked to think about how the content might relate to this case and whether it offers any solutions or strategies for assisting him.

Introduction

The nature of evidence has been the subject of considerable discussion. Whether you are a beginning practitioner or a senior clinician or even a manager of a health service organisation, the question of what constitutes appropriate evidence on which to base your practice is fundamental. For this reason it is a key element of the JBI Model of Evidence-Based Health Care, and it is the focus of this chapter.

Whenever health professionals engage in practice, they make numerous clinical decisions. In making such decisions, the practitioner draws on a wide range of knowledge. This will include knowledge of the basic biological and behavioural sciences; the health professional's assessment of the current context and of the individual patient; their own experience; and their own current understandings of research reports they may have recently read. All of the knowledge that is used to make a clinical decision can be referred to as evidence – and the validity of this evidence may be variable.

When making decisions, clinicians (often quite subconsciously) are frequently trying to select an appropriate activity or intervention and to assess the degree to which the decision will meet the four practice interests of health professionals; that is, the extent to which it is (Pearson, 2002):

- Effective in achieving the desired outcome.
- Appropriate for the place and time.
- Meaningful to the patient and her/his family and community.
- Feasible within the context of care and the resources available.

Thus, evidence for practice takes many forms, and relates to the four practice interests of health practitioners.

Feasibility, appropriateness, meaningfulness and effectiveness

The term 'evidence' is generally used to mean the basis of belief; the substantiation or confirmation that we need in order to believe that something is true. When used in relation to clinical practice, health professionals seek evidence to substantiate the worth of a very wide range of activities and interventions. This means that in each case the type of evidence needed will depend upon the nature of the activity and its purpose.

Feasibility

Feasibility is the extent to which an activity is **practical and practicable**. Clinical feasibility is about whether or not an activity or intervention is physically, culturally or financially practical or possible within a given context. In our smoking example, although an intervention such as nicotine replacement therapy may be effective and may even be appropriate, in low socio-economic populations it may not be feasible because of its costs. This may be compounded if smoking is both socially acceptable within the culture and less expensive.

In practice . . .

What would constitute evidence of feasibility in Joshua's case? What would be the implications of this for planning his care?

Appropriateness

Appropriateness is the extent to which an intervention or activity **fits with or is apt in a situation**. Clinical appropriateness is about how an activity or intervention relates to the context in which care is given. In the example of the effectiveness of the use of nicotine replacement therapy for smoking cessation, we may well find that it is effective in achieving the outcome of smoking cessation, but if we were interested in how appropriate such an intervention is for the client, we would be seeking to understand the cultural practices of the community in which the client lives. Evidence of appropriateness is best generated through the rigorous conduct of interpretative research with groups and communities.

In practice . . .

What would constitute evidence of appropriateness in Joshua's case? What would be the implications of this for planning his care?

Meaningfulness

Meaningfulness is the extent to which an intervention or activity is **experienced by the patient**. Meaningfulness relates to the personal experience, opinions, values, thoughts, beliefs, and interpretations of patients or clients.

In the example of the effectiveness of the smoking cessation intervention, while nicotine replacement therapy may be deemed an effective treatment, the individual attempting to quit may miss the physical involvement of their hands in the smoking process. This may impact on the effectiveness of nicotine patches. Evidence of meaningfulness is best generated through the rigorous conduct of interpretative research studies with patients.

In practice . . .

What would constitute evidence of meaningfulness in Joshua's case? What would be the implications of this for planning his care?

Effectiveness

Effectiveness is the extent to which an intervention, when used appropriately, achieves the **intended effect**. Clinical effectiveness is about the relationship between an intervention and clinical or health outcomes. Therefore, when seeking evidence of effectiveness, the focus is on the objective measurement of the effect of an intervention on specific outcomes. An example of evidence of effectiveness may be the demonstrated efficacy of all forms of nicotine replacement therapy in comparison with alternative treatments as the preferred first line treatment for achieving smoking cessation.

To establish the effect and effectiveness of this intervention on the outcome, the intervention must be administered in the same way for all of the subjects and the outcomes must also be measured in the same way. The most reliable approach to generating evidence of effectiveness is the conduct of a controlled clinical trial where patients are randomised to a treatment group or a control group; as many of the variables as possible are controlled so that only the effects of the intervention are likely to have led to the outcome, and quantitative measurements are compared using statistical techniques.

> **In practice . . .**
>
> What would constitute evidence of effectiveness in Joshua's case? What would be the implications of this for planning his care?

Of course there is more to evidence-based practice than just cause and effect! Decision-making revolves around many contributing factors, including evidence of feasibility, appropriateness and meaningfulness. What is required is appropriate methods for *translating* these different types of evidence into knowledge and information that is *meaningful* to practice!

The decision toolkit shown below illustrates the place and process of evidence in practice. This is intended to demonstrate that evidence is precisely that: it is a tool for clinicians to apply to achieve the best possible outcome for the patient.

Decision toolkit

Decision	Tools	Evaluation
What type of evidence is required to assist Joshua in his care and decision-making?	Patient assessment. Individualised approach to care.	Did the patient assessment and individualised approach to care result in the identification of the types of evidence required to assist Joshua?

Achieving a balance between evidence of effectiveness and other evidence interests for clinicians and consumers

The evidence-based practice movement has, until recently, focused largely on evidence of effectiveness. Pearson (1998) has argued that, while evidence-based practice includes an interest in research directed to the establishment of clinical effectiveness, it needs to go beyond this to include the qualitative domain. He says:

'Randomised trials are the gold standard for phenomena that we are interested in studying from a cause and effect perspective, but clearly they are not the gold standard if we are interested in how patients and nurses relate to each other, or if we are interested in how patients live through the experience of radiotherapy when they have a life-threatening illness. We have yet to work out how to assess the quality of alternative approaches to research other than the RCT.'

He goes on to suggest that 'evidence-based practice is not exclusively about effectiveness; it is about basing practice on the best available evidence'.

The diverse origins of problems in health care practice require a diversity of research methodologies. Thus, methodological approaches in this area need to be sufficiently eclectic to incorporate classical, medical and scientific designs along with the emerging qualitative and action-oriented approaches from the humanities and the social and behavioural sciences. The development of interdisciplinary research and a greater understanding of the relationship between medical, nursing and allied health interventions are also fundamental to the emergence of research methodologies that are relevant and sensitive to the health needs of consumers.

The nature of evidence

In general terms, evidence refers to data or information used to decide whether or not a claim or view should be trusted. In health care, practitioners and patients make numerous decisions and, in doing so, weigh up numerous types of information before taking action. Although the results of well-designed research are an obvious source of evidence, the results of formal research are by no means the only data used in everyday practice. Other determinants include the patient and his or her relevant others, the practitioner's own experiences and the nature and norms of the setting and culture in which the health care is being delivered. These are all rich sources of evidence to draw upon in making clinical decisions.

The dominant orthodoxy of regarding the results of quantitative research as evidence and all other knowledge as something other than evidence does not reflect the understanding of practice held by many clinicians. This is not surprising, given the nature and meaning of evidence in everyday life.

Evidence in its most generic sense has been defined as being 'the available facts, circumstances, etc. supporting or otherwise a belief, proposition, etc. or indicating whether a thing is true or valid'. Evidence in a legal sense has been defined as being 'information given personally or drawn from a document etc. and tending to prove a fact or proposition . . . or . . . statements or proofs admissible as testimony in a law court' (Pearsall and Trumball, 1995).

For philosophers, evidence is understood to be information bearing on the truth or falsity of a proposition. According to Audi (1995, p. 252):

'a person's evidence is generally taken to be all the information a person has, positive or negative, relevant to a proposition. The notion of evidence used in philosophy thus differs from the ordinary notion according to which physical objects, such as a strand

of hair or a drop of blood, counts as evidence. One's information about such objects could count as evidence in the philosophical sense.'

It is important, from a philosophical standpoint, to understand that the concept of evidence plays a key role in our understanding of knowledge and rationality. Traditionally, 'one has knowledge only when one has a true belief based on very strong evidence'. Moreover, for belief to be rational it must be based on adequate evidence, even when that evidence is insufficient to ground knowledge.

Evidence for health professionals

Some serious consideration has been given to the meaning of evidence in relation to the evidence-based health care movement. Dixon-Woods and Fitzpatrick (2001), for example, discuss the relevance of evidence elicited through qualitative research in systematic reviews, and Noblit and Hare (1998) describe how ethnographic approaches to inquiry generate evidence appropriate to practice.

According to Humphris (1999), the term 'evidence-based' in health care 'implies the use and application of research evidence as a basis on which to make health care decisions, as opposed to decisions not based on evidence'. Within the mainstream health field led by medicine and medical science, research has been narrowly confined to the empirico-analytical paradigm, focusing on objectivity, measurement and statistical significance. This process of knowledge generation involves testing a hypothesis or a set of hypotheses by deriving consequences from it and then testing whether those consequences hold true by experiment and observation. A theory of evidence assists here to the extent that it indicates what relationship should exist between the observation reports and the hypotheses if those reports are to constitute evidence for the hypotheses.

There is some legitimacy in regarding the randomised controlled trial, and other approaches that focus on measurement and statistical analysis, as the most desirable approach to evidence generation when the question relates to cause and effect relationships. However, health professionals have broader evidence interests that relate to the experience of health, illness and health care. Indeed, it is not unusual within the broad field of health care to find that the 'best available' evidence on a given topic cannot be reduced to a quantifiable value. Expert opinion – whether it is expressed by an individual, a learned body or a group of experts in the form of a consensus guideline – draws on the experience of practitioners. Well-designed qualitative research, while often not properly understood by researchers grounded in the physical sciences, constitutes 'good' human science.

Pearson (1999) argues for a pluralistic approach when considering 'what counts as evidence' for health care practices, and Evans and Pearson (2001) suggest that reviews that include qualitative evidence and/or quantitative evidence will be of importance to most practitioners. They go on to suggest, however, that 'optimal methods for reviewing qualitative research are still evolving'.

Although an obvious source of evidence is the results of well-designed research, such results are by no means the only data used in everyday practice. As previously indicated, the patient and her or his relevant others, the practitioner's own experiences, and the nature and norms of the setting and culture within which health care is being delivered are all rich sources of evidence upon which to draw in making clinical decisions.

In practice . . .

What forms of evidence would be of assistance in Joshua's case? Would you limit that evidence to that generated by relevant RCTs? If not, what sources of evidence would you accept? Where would you draw the line? Would expertise based on education and experience (i.e. opinion) suffice as evidence?

Expertise

Expertise is highly regarded among health care practitioners, and the possession of expertise is highly regarded too. It is essentially linked to the ability of a practitioner to 'have to hand' relevant information in a given area of practice. It is generally associated with the possession of large amounts of knowledge, and fluency in applying this knowledge. Expertise is difficult to quantify – and even more difficult to rank in terms of its reliability. However, a large proportion of health care practice relies on expertise. Practitioners who have expertise are titled experts, and the opinions of experts often represents the best available evidence in areas where research is limited, or where research on a specific question is difficult to conduct.

Experience

Experience is knowledge of and skill in something gained through being involved in or exposed to it over a period of time. It generally refers to know-how or procedural knowledge rather than propositional knowledge, and plays a major role in health care practice. When a practitioner makes a clinical decision, it is usual to weigh up external evidence with the practitioner's own experience. Thus, experience in itself is a source of evidence in health care practice.

Tradition

Tradition plays a major role in health care practices, largely because practitioners in all disciplines are required to participate in an extended period of education and training whereby they are socialised into the traditions of their profession and of the particular school and health services where they are educated. Tradition is an inherited pattern of thought or action that leads to a specific practice of long standing. Tradition may stem from logic and evidence from trial and error, but this is not generally the case.

Research

Although expertise and experience cannot be ignored as legitimate, internal sources of evidence for practice (and tradition can be seen as being not so legitimate), when the results of rigorous research are available, it is appropriate to weigh the results of external research against those internal sources of expertise, experience and tradition.

Evidence for health consumers

A significant trend in recent years has been the escalating interest of consumers of health care in the evidence-based movement. Increasingly, consumers are looking to the evidence to enable them to make more informed choices regarding their treatment and to more confidently discuss medical conditions and treatments, and to educate them regarding good health practices. There has been considerable debate regarding what should be considered evidence for health professionals, and while change is imminent, what is regarded as evidence for consumers remains uncertain.

Consumers have varying expectations and knowledge about evidence-based health care. However, it is evident that they too require not only information regarding effectiveness, but also information generated from qualitative research. It has been argued that qualitative information is important because consumers often have to make decisions about treatments and outcomes that are outside their own experience (NHMRC, 1999). Consumer information that recognises qualitative research may provide additional information regarding how people feel about their illness, how they experienced symptoms, how they coped and practical tips and advice that may not ordinarily be captured in quantitative-research-based consumer information. Qualitative research has an especially valuable role to play in answering questions that are not easily addressed exclusively by experimental methods. There are indeed areas where qualitative research alone is sufficient, or the only possible or desirable means of approaching a research question (Dixon-Woods and Fitzpatrick, 2001).

Where consumer-oriented health information is concerned, quantitative or qualitative research evidence is insufficient on its own. Consumers experience health-related problems directly and indirectly as individuals, family members or carers. Information regarding effectiveness is only one aspect of the diverse range of information they will require throughout the duration of that experience and the decision-making process involved. Therefore, methodological approaches in this area need to be eclectic enough to incorporate classical, medical and scientific designs and the emerging qualitative and action-oriented approaches from the humanities and social and behavioural sciences (Pearson, 2004). It is only in so doing that producers of evidence-based health information for consumers will accommodate effectively the various information requirements of consumers.

Just as health professionals have broader evidence interests that relate to the experience of health, illness and health care, so too do consumers. Pearson (1999,

2004) argues for a pluralistic approach when considering 'what counts as evidence' for health care practices and suggests that a process for systematic reviews that includes both qualitative evidence and quantitative evidence is necessary. It is suggested here that these two approaches are of equal importance to consumers of health care and provide a meaningful framework for decision-making.

Pearson (1998) argues that randomised trials are the gold standard for phenomena that we are interested in studying from a cause and effect perspective. However, they are not appropriate when attempting to illustrate to consumers the lived experience of a given treatment, therapy or procedure.

Conclusion

Historically, evidence of a quantitative nature has been considered to provide a stronger evidence base than qualitative methods. This narrow definition of what constitutes evidence for practice is problematic within the health care environment. While evidence of effectiveness of various interventions is necessary, it is evident that both health professionals and consumers require a range of information in order to facilitate change in practice and informed decision-making. The current climate is one that recognises the need to encompass evidence not only of effectiveness but also of feasibility, appropriateness and meaningfulness in order to achieve evidence-based health care practice.

In practice . . .

Think back to Joshua in the scenario at the beginning of this chapter and consider your approach to assisting him. Does the information in this chapter cause you to regard evidence differently? In the case of Joshua, how might you define what is meant by evidence of feasibility, appropriateness, meaningfulness and effectiveness?

Provide an example relevant to your specific profession and demonstrate the interplay between these different forms of evidence. Maybe it is similar to caring for someone like Joshua, or maybe you require different combinations of information types at different times. Reflect upon your experience as a health care professional in general terms and describe how evidence of feasibility, appropriateness, meaningfulness and effectiveness could impact on the decisions you make.

Further reading and resources

If you would like to know more about evidence for practice, the following may be of interest:

Humphris, D. (1999) Types of evidence. In: Harmer, S. and Collinson, G. (eds) *Achieving Evidence-based Practice: A Handbook for Practitioners*. London, Ballière Tindall.

Some useful resources for when thinking about evidence-based practice and the types of evidence available can be found at:

The Joanna Briggs Institute: www.joannabriggs.edu.au

Chapter 4

Health Care Evidence Generation

'Everything that can be counted does not necessarily count; everything that counts cannot necessarily be counted.' – Albert Einstein

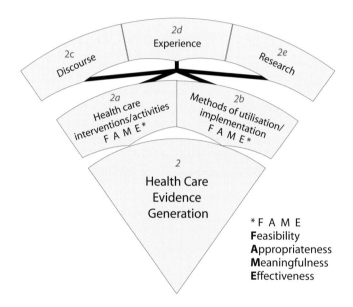

In Chapter 1 we explained the nature of evidence-based practice and the emergence and development of the evidence-based health care movement. In Chapter 2 we introduced the JBI Model of Evidence-based Health Care and its components. In Chapter 3 we examined the nature of evidence and the various types of evidence that we consider to be useful for informing practice. You should now have sufficient background information to enable you to make full use of the explanations of the components of the JBI Model in the remaining chapters of the book. We commence those explanations in Chapter 4 where we address that activity most fundamental to evidence-based practice, the generation of evidence. The basis of evidence-based practice is, of course, evidence. For this reason the generation of evidence is given pre-eminence both in its place at the top of the dial of the clock and because, in terms of process, it is first in time.

This chapter discusses:

- The generation of evidence through research.
- Quantitative and qualitative research approaches.

- How different research approaches address the evidence interests of health professionals.

In practice . . .

A client who has been receiving treatment for lung cancer is transferred to your care. Skye has been smoking since she was a young girl, and although she is aware that she needs to quit, previous attempts have proved unsuccessful. She has heard that acupuncture can work for people trying to quit smoking and asks you for some information. Your supervisor suggests that you conduct a search to find information regarding the effectiveness of acupuncture for smoking cessation. In order to gather this type of information, you first need to establish the type of research that would identify best practice regarding effectiveness.

As you read through this chapter, keep in mind Skye's situation. At various points you will be asked to think about how the content might relate to this case and whether it offers any solutions or strategies for assisting her.

Introduction

Evidence for health care is generated through research, experience and the formulation of opinion. Research is essentially the systematic search for truth or knowledge. As such, it is of fundamental importance to the beginning practitioner who must cultivate the habit of ensuring that their practice is supported by the best available evidence generated by research. For the advanced practitioner it is a critical mechanism for the improvement of practice. Often the advanced practitioner is dealing with intractable problems that necessitate further research to improve outcomes for their patients/clients. It is frequently the advanced practitioners who are in the best position to conduct that research.

At still another level, the managers of health service organisations will be concerned to identify those interventions and practices that produce optimal outcomes for patients/clients in the most efficient and cost-effective manner. The process of identifying those interventions and practices involves research, and again, the managers may well be best positioned, if not to actually conduct the research, to commission it.

It will be clear from this account that all of us who are involved in the provision of health care have a vested interest in knowing not just how to locate research but also how to evaluate research and even how to conduct good-quality research. It is patently the case that much research is conducted that we may not consider to be good quality.

An enterprise so fundamental as research is, of necessity, the subject of much scrutiny, debate and opinion. There are therefore a wide range of views and perspectives on what constitutes 'good' research, how varying research approaches can be classified, and how the research process can best be understood and communicated. This systematic search for truth or knowledge provides us with the evidence on which to ground our health care practice. In this chapter we endeavour to provide you with a 'mud map' of research approaches along with their significance and relationship to the evidence for practice that is generated through research.

The debates about the nature of knowledge and research have given rise to a number of different approaches to research. The existence of these various approaches makes it essential for those who aspire to evidence-based practice to at least familiarise themselves with the variety of approaches, because while there is debate about the relative worth of different approaches, the different approaches have evolved to answer different types of questions.

Since the emergence of modern science in the eighteenth century, health professionals have pursued a number of different pathways to develop their work (clinical practice) and to generate knowledge (medical, nursing and health science). Science is systematically developed knowledge and is advancing rapidly internationally in the health field as health professionals increasingly engage in research.

Our view of what constitutes 'good' science and 'good' research-based evidence has almost certainly come about as a result of the historical development of western thought, as well as our own experiences of the world and the total context of our experience. The overall view of the world shaped by these kinds of influences leads, in the case of research, to a conviction of what does and does not constitute the true picture and of how one can legitimately search for truth, knowledge or evidence. Such convictions are often referred to as paradigms.

Guiding paradigms in research

Chinn and Jacobs (1987) define a paradigm as 'a generally accepted world view or philosophy, a structure within which the theories of the discipline are organised'.

A paradigm consists of the basic beliefs about the phenomena that concern a discipline. Broad, philosophical paradigms, suggests Botha (1989), give rise to assumptions in disciplinary groups that quite profoundly influence practice, research and theory. Chessick (1980) asserts that 'it is very important to realise that much in our conclusions about anything comes not from the study of things but from the philosophical decisions implicit in the way we start'.

Allen et al. (1986) describe three prevailing paradigms that are generally adhered to in western thought and scholarship – the positivist, the interpretive and the critical. It would be wrong to assume that this is an all-inclusive categorisation of guiding paradigms, of course, but it is of use to consider these three classes of approach.

The positivist paradigm

Positivism (that is, logical positivism, or the empirico-analytical paradigm) attempts to view the world objectively in order to manipulate it. Fay (1975) says that the positivist stance attempts to:

*'understand a state of affairs scientifically only to the extent that we have knowledge
of what to do in order to control it, and it is thus that the ability to control phenomena provides the framework in terms of which scientific explanation proceeds.'*

Consequently, knowledge is generated through the use of controlled observation
and experimentation in an attempt to confirm explanations. The researcher starts
off with a theoretical idea, which is then transformed into a hypothesis to be
tested using objective methods. If the hypothesis is confirmed, it is then assumed
that this will occur in the same way in the future and thus the event and its
results become predictable. Many areas of knowledge of interest to health professionals are amenable to such an approach, especially those that relate to physiological processes.

The positivist paradigm is concerned with quantitative theory, which aims
at control. In order to maintain objectivity, distance between the research
process/researcher and the research subject(s) is meticulously maintained. The
central approach of the positivist paradigm is deductive in that theory is developed and then tested. If it is supported through testing it becomes 'fact', which
is generalisable when the same events occur in the future.

The positivist position has a long history in western thought and is by far the
most common approach in the health sciences. Its beginnings can be traced to
Plato and Aristotle, and its real emergence as a school of thought can be seen in
the work of Descartes and Newton. The powerful influence of the early philosophers on contemporary thought should not be underestimated. A great deal of
western culture and intellectual life is still heavily laden with the views of the
human condition that have evolved from the philosophers of the past. Western
health care systems value the positivist paradigm highly, with some health professionals regarding this approach as the only legitimate framework for health
research.

It is obvious that research based on the positivist paradigm has served human-
ity well, having uncovered numerous explanations for phenomena in the physical world that were previously mysterious. This is especially evident in the area
of medical science. Thus, it should not be devalued or dismissed lightly in areas
of study that are amenable to control and measurement and where causality can
reasonably be identified. However, the use of positivism to examine social
aspects of human life and the lived experience does not always fit so well.

The positivist paradigm has been subjected to vigorous critique for over a
century, yet it still remains dominant in western thought. Critiquing positivism
has become almost passé – it has been a part of intellectual debate for centuries,
yet its credibility is still relatively strong. The two central problems of the positivist tradition that have concerned its critics are:

- Its reduction of the universe to mechanistic systems and structures.
- Its mistaken assumption that objectivity is reality.

The positivist paradigm has as its goal the separation of reality from subjectivity. 'Truth' is seen to be unambiguous and not open to interpretation
and valid knowledge is assumed to be unaffected by contextual or situational

contingencies. Structures are seen to be objective and able to be studied without recourse to the personal experiences of the people who are perceived to be regulated by the structures. In this way structures have been reified and divorced from the actions of people (Bauman, 1978). Researchers are seen to be 'neutral observers' (Winstead-Fry, 1980, p. 3).

The social world is perceived as being orderly and as acting on the individual – regulating actions and ensuring stability (Munhall and Oiler, 1986, p. xiii). Behaviour and verbal responses have been studied in isolation from interpretation and meaning. Research informed by this tradition is concerned with prediction, control and generalisability. Such research relies upon quantitative methods, and results are usually reported in numerical form following statistical analysis.

In the past, clinical researchers, in response to studies in research, the philosophy of science and other disciplines, have tended to adopt entrenched positions on either side of the qualitative/quantitative divide or according to the positivist/interpretive/critical categorisation of the pursuit of knowledge. Characterising the categorisations of research in these two different ways has significant implications for understanding research paradigms, which are explained later in this chapter. At this point it is important to appreciate the need to be sufficiently balanced and open in our views to recognise the role of quantification and experiment in research on the human body and the effects of interventions on treating disease and illness. A balanced position also demands, however, an understanding of the role of other approaches to researching the human condition that pursue questions of meaning, individual and social action, and the processes of living in the world.

We have already mentioned two alternative social science paradigms, which stem from views quite different to those of positivism. The interpretive and critical paradigms are certainly worthy of further examination in the current context.

In the interpretive paradigm, theory is inductive (i.e. moves from specific observations to more general conceptualisations) and is concerned with exposing implicit meaning. Unlike the deductive processes of the quantitative approach, which is aimed at measurement and control, the interpretive paradigm seeks to achieve understanding.

The critical paradigm, like the interpretive, is inductive but it has as its aim the emancipation of knowledge and practice. It is concerned with the relationship between meaning and the social notions of autonomy and responsibility.

These two alternatives to the positivist paradigm have much to offer health care in clarifying our understandings about the nature of our clients and about our practice. In researching health care, questions can be pursued from a paradigmatic stance that is appropriate if the positivist position is seen as just one alternative rather than the only legitimate way to do research. The determining factor as to the appropriate research paradigm for a given project should be the research question itself, rather than any personal predilection on the part of the researcher for a particular paradigm.

Our ability to view the evolving relationship between research and practice clearly is dependent upon our understandings of research in its broadest sense.

In practice . . .

Would the positivist paradigm offer any possibility of generating evidence that would be of assistance to Skye in determining whether acupuncture could assist her in quitting smoking? If so, can you suggest how it might do so?

The interpretive paradigm

The interpretive paradigm is grounded on assumptions and methods that are very different to those of positivism. Its foundations are credited to the sociologist-philosopher Alfred Schutz who argued for a distinction between the natural sciences and the social sciences.

Rather than using objective, quantifiable methods to gather information, the interpretive stance involves listening to people or watching what they do and using the human imagination and understandings of those participating in order to interpret their meanings. True knowledge is dependent upon whether or not the participants accept those meanings, rather than on whether they will identify cause, predict outcome, or allow control (Fay, 1975).

The theorist builds up theory on the basis of the understandings that arise out of the people studied, rather than testing hypotheses. Theory is seen as 'a skeletal, deprived view of reality that is drawn from everyday practical activity and knowledge' (Allen, Benner et al., 1986). Theory is not generalisable, and is used in order to understand. Essentially, theory is seen as being already embedded in practice, although not made explicit.

Research and the subjective human world are seen to be inextricably linked, and formal theory (i.e. that which is documented and accessible but derived from knowledge embedded in experience of the world) is used to guide the novice but is transformed and refined by the expert.

In practice . . .

How useful would the interpretive paradigm be in offering guidance to Skye in determining whether acupuncture could assist her in quitting smoking? How might this paradigm be useful in this situation?

The critical paradigm

The critical paradigm goes beyond the boundaries of the positivist and interpretive paradigms. It seeks to generate theory from action or practice in order to help people address change in the interests of social justice, and therefore unambiguously integrates research and practice. The researcher-practitioner aims at raising consciousness, both their own and that of others, through collaboratively analysing and seeking understandings of the real situation, and searching out alternative ways of seeing the situation. This paradigm involves a dialectic transaction between research and practice, and therefore welds the two together. It focuses on theory in action or action theory. This perspective, argues Allen (1985), offers health professionals the opportunity to translate frequently voiced rhetoric about the interrelationship between research and practice into the real world of practice.

(Note: Dialectic refers to a process whereby one explores ideas through confronting contradictions and searching for ways to resolve these contradictions or to explain them. This is an important concept in interpretive and critical research.)

The qualitative/quantitative debate

Currently there is a tendency to classify research as quantitative or qualitative. Just as our description of three prevailing paradigms are classifications of approaches to research, so too is the quantitative/qualitative terminology. An alternative is to use the terms qualitative and quantitative in relation to data and method. While the positivist paradigm essentially focuses on quantification, this does not exclude quantifying qualitative data. For example, a survey of opinions on an issue (which would consist of qualitative data) can be analysed by counting how many times particular opinions are expressed and then applying statistical tests. Similarly, quantitative data may be appropriate in critical research. In discussing the quantitative/qualitative debate we are therefore confining our thoughts to quantitative/qualitative data and wish to avoid using these terms to describe overall, broad approaches to research.

Qualitative versus quantitative data

Qualitative data is collected in order to derive understanding of phenomena from a subjective perspective. The focus is on description, understanding and empowerment. Where theory is developed it is based on inductive reasoning, and is grounded in reality as it is perceived and experienced by the participants involved.

Conversely, quantitative data is collected in order to control phenomena. The focus is on theory-testing and prediction and control. Theory derived from previous research is used to formulate a hypothesis or testable idea. Based on the process of deduction, the hypothesis is then tested using objective methods.

The relative merits of both of these forms of data are the subject of much heated debate in the health care system. On the one hand, qualitative methods are seen to most certainly increase understanding but they are often criticised as 'biased' and subjected to the question 'Well, now that we understand, so what?' On the other hand, quantitative methods are seen to give an apparently unbiased, objective picture of a situation or phenomenon, but they are often criticised as being 'only half the story' or of being overly concerned with numbers and statistics.

Central to the debate, however, must be the paradigmatic stance from which the researcher works, and the stance from which the consumer of research reads.

As long as the method is consistent with, or true to, the paradigm that underpins the research, and as long as it is an appropriate method to address the research question, in theory the debate becomes redundant. However, the debate still continues to rage largely because of deeply entrenched allegiances to a particular paradigm.

Paradigm, methodology and method

As you will by now have worked out, the paradigmatic stance one takes influences the research methodology one then selects as a basis for a research study. Similarly, the methodological position adopted influences the way in which data is collected. The processes of data collection and analysis – the methods – are also dependent upon the methodology adopted (Table 4.1).

The three paradigms discussed in this chapter are associated with a range of methodological approaches, which are consistent with the philosophical view of knowledge embodied in each paradigm.

The quantitative research approach

Quantitative research approaches are characterised by an adherence to a set of sequential steps to acquire dependable data. The major broad designs are experimental, descriptive and correlational designs. Experimental design is usually regarded as the 'gold standard' and the central concern of experimental research

Table 4.1 Paradigms, methodologies and methods for research studies.

Paradigm	Methodology	Methods
Positivist paradigm	Randomised controlled trials	Methods that measure outcomes such as temperature, blood pressure, attitudes, etc.
	Cohort studies	Methods that measure outcomes (as above)
	Case series studies	Methods that measure outcomes (as above)
	Time series studies	Methods that measure outcomes (as above)
Interpretive paradigm	Phenomenology	Interviews
	Historiography	Textual analysis; interviews
	Ethnography	Participant observation; interviews of key informants
	Grounded theory	Participant observation; interviews
Critical paradigm	Action research	Participative group interaction; observation; interviews
	Feminist research	Participative group interaction; observation; interviews

is to determine cause–effect relationships. Within health care, experimental and quasi-experimental research is warranted when the researcher wants to establish what effect an intervention or activity has on specified outcomes. The researcher using these approaches therefore sets out to introduce or manipulate a variable (i.e. any attribute of a person or object that varies or changes its value), rather than (as in non-experimental work) gathering data on what is observed or measured without changing practices or interventions. The randomised, controlled trial is an example of experimental research.

Fundamental to experimental research are three central features:

- Introducing or manipulating the intervening variable
- Controlling other variables
- Randomising into experimental and control groups

Quasi-experimental research – often used in nursing and allied health – tries to comply with these features as much as possible but some of the true features of an experiment may not be possible: for example, the sample may not be randomised. Examples of quasi-experimental design are time series designs (both multiple and interrupted) where the approach is to identify trends before and after the introduction of an intervention; cross-sectional design (which looks at data at a single point in time); and case study design.

The interpretive research approach

Phenomenological thought, in its broader sense, is the philosophy that underpins all interpretive methodologies. Within the phenomenological tradition a number of different methodological approaches have been developed, and although phenomenology as a philosophical stance informs all of these perspectives, it also forms one particular methodology.

Phenomenological philosophy

Phenomenological philosophy is grounded in the view that 'what people say and do [is] a product of how they define their world' (Taylor and Bogdan, 1984, pp. 8–9).

How people define their world is related to:

- The interactions they have with others
- How they perceive others to perceive them
- The ways in which they have learned to deal with life experiences, good and bad
- The amount of perceived control they have, and the significance to them of perceived control

Reality is not a static given, nor is it some 'fact' or 'truth'. Rather it is a social construct (Berger and Luckman, 1971), which is always in the process of being constructed and negotiated. What was considered a truth or reality at one time can be interpreted quite differently in another place, at another time, or in another context. Individuals and their environments are therefore in a constant and reflexive relationship.

From this perspective, human beings do not merely reflect the social processes that prevail; they actively construct social processes and relations by creating others through their evaluations of them and by helping to create and project their own personae or self-images. The social process is therefore seen as dialectical. Neither the self nor society should be seen as derivative of the other as in a cause and effect relationship. Rather, both may be thought of as mutually constitutive (Starr, 1982, p. 259).

Phenomenology

As well as being the philosophical base of the interpretive paradigm, phenomenology has also emerged as a specific methodological approach for research. Phenomenological methodology is concerned with discovering the 'essence' of experience. It asks the question 'What is it like to have that experience?'

Ethnography

Ethnography is basically the study of culture. It asks the question 'What is the way of life of this group of people and what does it mean?' and it recognises everyday life as an ongoing achievement worthy of study. Like phenomenology, ethnography has become increasingly popular in nursing and health research as nurses and other health professionals attempt to understand the contexts of both health care systems and the communities that they serve.

Grounded theory

Grounded theory is the generation of theory that is grounded in the real world. It asks the question 'What social processes are occurring here and what do they mean?' through searching for and generating theoretical explanations of what is occurring in a social setting. The grounded theory approach aims at systematically collecting and analysing data in such a way that theory emerges and is developed from the data. In other words, data is not constrained to fit some predetermined theoretical framework; rather, the data itself defines the boundaries and directs theorising. It is based on symbolic interactionist theory and was developed largely by Glaser and Strauss (1967).

The critical research approach

The critical paradigm moves beyond the interpretive. The interpretive approach aims at describing and understanding; the critical approach incorporates this aim, but as well as asking what is happening, it asks why and explores change and emancipation. Critical researchers seek to question why things are as they are and to generate change through bringing problems or injustices forward for conscious debate and consideration. Critical approaches involve working with people collaboratively to analyse and seek out understandings of the real situation, and to search out alternative ways of seeing the situation. The central focus is on the emancipation of knowledge and practice.

Critical theory

The development of critical theory is most closely associated with the philosopher Jurgen Habermas. In his book *Knowledge and Human Interests* (1971), Habermas says that there are three areas of knowledge that are integral to human existence:

- Technical interest (which equates with the goals and processes of the positivist paradigm)
- Practical interest (which equates with the goals and processes of the interpretive paradigm)
- Emancipatory interest (which equates with the goals and processes of the critical paradigm)

These three knowledge interests underpin methodological approaches to the generation of knowledge and shape what we regard as knowledge as well as the procedures for discovering and legitimating knowledge.

Technical interest

The technical interest is concerned with the ability of individuals to control and manipulate their environment in order to survive (Bernstein, 1986). This ability has given rise to the positivist tradition.

Positivism is technical in as much as it pursues mechanistic explanations of human action. It is not rejected by critical theorists but it is seen as only one area of knowledge and not, as is often claimed, the standard by which all knowledge should be measured.

Practical interest

Practical interest is concerned with human interaction and the inter-subjective meanings of social activity. The interpretive paradigm is based in practical interest and aims at the clarification of inter-subjective understanding rather than technical control and manipulation. Practical knowledge is knowledge of self and others through shared meaning.

Emancipatory interest

Emancipatory interest is concerned with self-knowledge generated through self-reflection. It is based on the human capacity to act rationally, to reason self-consciously, and to make decisions in the light of available knowledge, rules and needs. Habermas's 'emancipatory interest' is an interest in reason, an interest in controlling the use of technical knowledge and in directing actions towards the realisation of personal, social and professional goals.

The critical paradigm and research methodology

From this critical view, the individual's consciousness of self is produced by perception of the relationships developed with others and by the conditions (structures) that enhance or constrain action. In this way the politics of change can be seen for what they are – the development within the individual of a commitment to an already existing professional culture and socialised structure. From this socially critical perspective, research can be seen as a political process.

The critical paradigm focuses on action and sees this as legitimate, respectable and worthy of trust. While adherents of positivism can, and do, cite several philosophical viewpoints as foundations for legitimising positivist methods, critical theorists also cite a variety of different philosophical viewpoints that legitimise critical methods.

Action research

Action research is the pursuit of knowledge through working collaboratively on describing the social world and acting on it in order to change it. Through acting on the world in this way, critical theory and understandings are generated. Action research asks the question 'What is happening here and how could it be different?'

Action research involves reflecting on the world in order to achieve change and then entering into a cyclical process of reflection, changing and evaluating. It is based on a number of important concepts, with which you should become familiar. Those concepts are:

- *Praxis* – that is, the art of acting upon the conditions 'one faces' in order to change them. It was Aristotle who first articulated praxis, and contrasted it to theora, which is comprised of those sciences and activities concerned with knowing for its own sake, arguing that they were two necessary dimensions of a truly human and free life.
- *Hermeneutics* – a concept originally concerned with the interpretation of writing. The hermeneutical circle argues that no knowledge is possible without presuppositions. In the social sciences, the hermeneutical circle takes the form of attempting an initial holistic understanding of a social system and then using this understanding as a basis for interpreting parts of the system. Knowledge is gained dialectically by proceeding from the whole to its parts and then back again. Each time an incongruence occurs between the part and the whole, a re-conceptualisation takes place.
- *Critical theory* – as indicated earlier, this rests on the premise that theory is embedded in action, so that what is to count as truth will be partially determined by specific ways in which theory relates to practical action.

It will be readily apparent from the description of action research that the three concepts of praxis, hermeneutics and critical theory are of fundamental importance for this research methodology.

Feminist research

Feminist methodology is broad in scope and approach. It is based on the assumption that feminine thought and action is oppressed by the dominant masculine paradigm. It seeks to value the experiences and actions of women through the use of collaborative feminist processes.

Feminist theories have attempted to redress the male bias operant in most research. Stanley and Wise (1983, p. 35) argue that most feminist theory has also been developed within the dominant paradigm and has not questioned the ways in which such knowledge is constituted. Language and its relationship to what counts as knowledge and the social construction of the scientific paradigm have been treated as non-problematic. Additionally, or perhaps consequently, women's oppression has been blamed upon 'the system', whether this be capitalism or patriarchy. Women are thus viewed as passive and acted upon, rather than active agents negotiating their realities. Feminist theories have been categorised according to 'types' (e.g. Marxist, liberal, radical and so on).

More recently feminist theorists have begun to recognise the disjunction between feminist beliefs and the dominant paradigm. Reflecting this recognition has been the increasing association between feminist research and interpretive and critical methodologies. There is, for instance, a contradiction between believing that the personal is the political (that is, the views and feelings of an individual are just as important as the dominant or majority view) and positivist philosophy.

There is a further problem in undertaking research that assumes the subjective is a variable to be discounted, and that the researcher's interpretation is more 'truthful' and valid than that of the researched when one is arguing for the empowerment of women. There is an inconsistency in arguing for the empowerment of women and researching within a paradigm that places the researched in a subordinate position. Recognising these inconsistencies and contradictions, many researchers are now espousing collaboration in the researcher-researched relationship (e.g. Oakley, 1981; MacPherson, 1983; Cannon, 1989).

Also consistent with feminist ideology is the recognition given by critical theory to the reflexive relationship existing between the research and the researcher (Schwartz and Jacobs, 1979, p. 360). The critical approach legitimises the recognition and explication of biases. Stanley and Wise (1983, p. 49) articulate the obvious:

> '[Not doing research] is the only way that the researcher's self can be excluded from the centre of the research process . . . it is impossible both to experience and not to experience, to do research and not to do research through the medium of one's conscious-

ness . . . this consciousness and experience should be made explicit within the research.'

In contrast to traditional approaches, this recognises the impact of the researcher upon the negotiation of meaning within the research situation, and rather than pretending a purity contingent upon detachment, it defines the researcher as part of the research.

Different types of evidence are generated from different types of research. It is important to be able to identify which research results in these different types of evidence in order to be able to produce *meaningful* information upon which to base practice.

Decision toolkit

Decision	Tools	Evaluation
Need to establish the type of research that would identify best practice regarding effectiveness.	A solid understanding of research paradigms is required to make this assessment.	Has the research identified provided Skye with an applicable and appropriate answer to her question?

Sources for evidence of feasibility

Evidence of feasibility can come from a number of different sources. The results of well-designed cultural studies can inform decisions related to feasibility from a contextual perspective. The results of economic studies are appropriate in establishing feasibility from a cost/resource perspective. Research that uses participative methods that seek to understand how specific interventions or activities are accepted and implemented by practitioners or patients can generate results that are appropriate evidence when considering the feasibility of introducing a change in practice.

Sources for evidence of appropriateness

The results of well-designed interpretive studies that focus on culture and social relationships and other forms of research that use methods that generate understandings of social beliefs, values and norms represent appropriate evidence for practitioners when they need to make a judgement about the appropriateness of an intervention or activity (Pearson, 2004). The appropriateness of an activity or intervention, or the social meaning of a phenomenon, can only be understood through the conduct of research that attempts to interpret social norms. Ethnographic and grounded theory approaches are examples of research relevant to this interest.

Sources for evidence of meaningfulness

The results of well-designed interpretive research and other forms of research that use methods that allow for the development of understandings of what a phenomenon means to individuals represent appropriate evidence for practitioners when they need to make a judgement about the meaningfulness of a phenomenon, intervention or activity (Pearson, 2004). The meanings arising out of patients' experiences of an illness, an intervention or a specific phenomenon such as pain can only be understood through the conduct of research that seeks to capture the experiences of patients and, through interpretation, to explicate these meanings. Phenomenology is an approach that is often used to elicit this type of evidence.

Sources for evidence of effectiveness

The results of well-designed clinical trials and other forms of research that use methods that allow for the assessment of the statistical significance of the results represent strong evidence for practitioners when they need to make a judgement about the effectiveness of a treatment or intervention (Dawes et al., 1999, p. 3). The effectiveness of a drug or surgical procedure, or of the use of specific exercises, dressings or physical restraints on specified outcomes can only be established through the conduct of research that attempts to control the variables to the extent that the effect found can be attributed to a specific intervention. The results of cohort/survival studies represent appropriate evidence related to prognosis, and the results of cohort or case control studies are appropriate sources of evidence when considering risk.

Conclusion

As we have discussed in earlier chapters, 'evidence' is the data or information we use to decide whether or not a claim or view should be trusted. Evidence-based practice promotes the application of research evidence as a basis on which to make health care decisions. Although expert opinion and experience can be legitimately regarded as sources of evidence, the results of rigorous research (which sometimes draws on expertise and experience) represent a 'higher level' of evidence because the discipline involved in conducting research – regardless of the paradigmatic stance adopted – makes the process of generating the evidence sufficiently explicit for us to determine the degree to which the evidence is valid.

Health professionals will always, to some degree, base some elements of their practice on evidence arising out of experience or from acknowledged experts; this is partly because there will always be gaps in the research evidence and partly because, even if strong external research-based evidence exists, clinical judgement involves weighing this evidence against the context of care, the needs of the patient and the practitioner's own knowledge. Central to professional practice is a commitment to making clinical decisions that are informed by the best available evidence.

In practice . . .

Skye's interest in acupuncture as an intervention for smoking cessation is similar to many cases that occur in the clinical environment every day. Regardless of whether such a search for information is initiated by a consumer, another health professional or your own personal interest, it is important to understand the types of information that are generated from different types of research.

In your own words, describe the three research paradigms outlined in this chapter, then choose an intervention of specific interest to you and see if you can identify examples of sources of evidence of feasibility, appropriateness, meaningfulness and effectiveness. Think about how these types of information might impact on practice and your own clinical decision-making (both as a health professional and as a consumer).

Further reading and resources

If you are interested in learning more about the material addressed in this chapter, we would suggest the following sources:

Australian Science and Technology OnThe Internet: www.nla.gov.au/oz/sciencew.html

Cody, W. K. and Mitchell, G. J. (2002) Nursing knowledge and human science revisited: practical and political considerations. *Nursing Science Quarterly* 1.

Guba, E. G. and Lincoln, Y. S. (1994) Competing paradigms in qualitative research. In: Denzin, N. K. and Lincoln, Y. S. (eds) *Handbook of Qualitative Research*, pp. 105–17. Thousand Oaks, CA, Sage.

National Information Center on Health Services Research and Health Care Technology (NICHSR): www.nlm.nih.gov/nichsr/hsrsites.html

Chapter 5

Evidence Synthesis: The Systematic Review

'The hundreds of hours spent conducting a scientific study ultimately contributes only a piece of an enormous puzzle. The value of any single study is derived from how it fits with and expands previous work, as well as from the study's intrinsic properties. Through systematic review the puzzle's intricacies may be disentangled.' – C.D. Mulrow

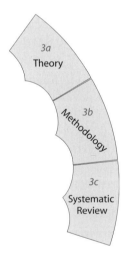

This chapter sees the clock tick around from the generation of evidence to the synthesis of evidence. Theory and methodology are important elements here because of the need to establish the validity of the process. However, the main tool of evidence synthesis is the systematic review, and this is the vehicle for demonstrating and explaining the theory and methodology employed. This is very much a 'how to' chapter that will show you how to conduct a systematic review and it will also assist reviewers in examining their approach to evidence review.

This chapter discusses:

- The purpose of systematically reviewing the evidence.
- Developing a systematic review protocol.
- Searching for the evidence.
- Selecting appropriate studies from the search results.

In practice . . .

Harry is an asthmatic adolescent who, regardless of his parent's tireless efforts to stop him from smoking, continues to smoke because 'all of his mates do'. He has been admitted to hospital after suffering yet another serious asthma attack and his parents are distraught, having tried every strategy known to them. You are aware that significant research exists on different strategies for smoking cessation but much of it is conflicting and you need to be certain of the information you provide. How do you make an accurate assessment of the information available and decide what to base your practice on?

   As you read through this chapter, keep in mind Harry's situation. At various points you will be asked to think about how the content might relate to this case and whether it offers any solutions or strategies for assisting him.

Introduction

In previous chapters we have introduced the idea of evidenced-based health care and considered the introduction and development of evidenced-based practice. These were 'big picture' chapters that necessitated a consideration of evidence, and what evidence might be suitable for informing health care practice. This in turn led us to an examination of what is meant by research, along with the various perspectives and paradigms that have evolved in relation to research. These are the mechanisms through which evidence is generated. Through this discussion we have emphasised the need for identifying relevant research on a topic and for appraising or evaluating that evidence. Now we have come to the point of bringing the research together to distil and synthesise the evidence. In short, we have come to the tools of the EBHC trade, and chief among these is the systematic review.

   Understanding the systematic review process is central to understanding the modus operandi of the EBHC model. You will see as you work your way through this chapter that a full systematic review is a major undertaking. You will also see, however, how useful these reviews can be. You may want to be involved in the conduct of reviews on a major scale or on a more modest level in order to answer questions that you have that are specific to your speciality. Either way, you will find that in this chapter, where we concentrate on the first phase of the systematic review (i.e. locating the evidence), and the next, where we deal with appraisal of evidence, there is enough practical guidance to enable you to become involved in conducting a review.

   The systematic review process is a fundamental component of evidence-based practice. Busy practitioners rarely have the opportunity to engage in the generation and conduct of systematic reviews in isolation, and thus there are a large number of groups across the world that facilitate this process. There are also a growing number of specialist collaborations, institutes and centres with skilled staff employed to train systematic reviewers, conduct systematic reviews and facilitate collaboration between reviewers.

   The nature of systematic reviews is changing and in recent years significant progress has been made toward broadening the scope of what evidence may be included (as discussed in previous chapters). The initial phase of a systematic review is fundamentally important to the success of the review. Every effort should be made during this phase to ensure that a good-quality review in the field of interest does not already exist and that none is in progress. This is a 'how to' chapter that will assist reviewers in ensuring that the quality of their review is of the highest.

Overview of the systematic review process

The systematic review is a form of research; indeed, it is frequently referred to as 'secondary research'. Primary research involves the design and conduct of a study, including the collection of primary data from patients and clients, and its analysis and interpretation. The systematic review also collects and analyses data – but usually from published and unpublished reports of completed research. Thus, the systematic reviewer uses secondary sources of data.

As in any research endeavour, the first step in the systematic review is the development of a proposal or protocol. Protocol development begins with an initial search of databases such as the Cochrane Database of Systematic Reviews and Database of Abstracts of Reviews of Effects (DARE) to establish whether or not a recent review report exists. The Cochrane database can be accessed via http://www.cochrane.org while the DARE database can be found at http://www.york.ac.uk/inst/crd/darehp.htm.

If the topic has not been the subject of a systematic review, a review protocol is developed.

The review question

As with any research, it is important to have a clear question. The protocol should state in detail the questions or hypotheses that will be pursued in the review. Questions should be specific regarding, for example, the consumers, setting, interventions or phenomena and outcomes to be investigated. This will vary according to the purpose of the review. When a review focuses on the effect of an intervention on specific outcomes or on prognosis, diagnosis or risk, precise descriptions of the interventions and outcomes are required. If the review is more concerned with the evidence on the subjective experience of a phenomenon, activity or intervention, outcomes may be less specific.

Example for a quantitative review on smoking cessation:

The effectiveness of acupuncture and associated techniques for the achievement of smoking cessation (think back to Skye's case in Chapter 4).

Example for a qualitative review on smoking cessation:

The experience of pregnant women attempting to quit smoking.

In practice . . .

Think about Harry's case now. What would be an appropriate review question to locate evidence that may be of assistance to him in quitting smoking?

The review protocol

As in any research endeavour, the development of a rigorous research proposal or protocol is vital for a high-quality systematic review. Systematic reviewers develop a protocol that is subjected to peer review before they commence the review (for example, Cochrane Collaboration review protocols are approved by a relevant Cochrane Review Group before the review commences and JBI review protocols are approved by JBI before commencement). Once a protocol is finalised, it is lodged in an online database so that other reviewers interested in a given topic can search these databases to avoid duplication of reviews (to view an example protocol, see Appendix 1).

The review protocol provides a predetermined plan to ensure scientific rigour and minimise potential bias. It also allows for periodic updating of the review if necessary. Updating systematic reviews is imperative in a climate of continuous information production. New research knowledge is generated on a regular basis and therefore regular updates of systematic reviews are essential in order to ensure that health practices are based on the most current research evidence. It is generally accepted that this will occur on a three- to five-year cycle, or as deemed necessary (depending on the topic).

A number of decisions critical to the quality of the systematic review need to be made at this point and it is important that the protocol reflects this. It is important to bear in mind at this point the discussion in Chapter 3 of the different approaches to research. It will be obvious that where a systematic review seeks to utilise multiple forms of research, the review criteria will be different from those associated with a review using research involving only quantitative data. However, regardless of whether the intention is to conduct a review of effectiveness, a review of qualitative research or a comprehensive systematic review that includes multiple types of research evidence, there are standard criteria that should be addressed in the protocol.

Every effort should be made to adhere to the criteria set in the protocol although, as with primary research, there may be instances where changes are unavoidable. Any such changes should be declared in the final review report.

Learning activity

Think of your particular field of interest and develop a question that you are interested in answering. Be as specific and definitive as possible, trying to include in your question details of the population, interventions, comparisons and outcomes of interest. Now keep this question in mind as you work through this chapter.

Title:	
Background:	
Objectives:	
Criteria for considering studies for this review:	Types of participants:
	Types of intervention:
	Types of outcome measures:
	Types of studies:
Search strategy for identification of studies:	
Methods of the review:	Selecting studies for inclusion:
	Assessment of quality:
	Methods used to collect data from included studies:
	Methods used to synthesise data:
	Date review to commence:
	Date review to complete:

Fig. 5.1 The Joanna Briggs Institute Review Protocol (reproduced with the permission of the Joanna Briggs Institute).

An example of a review protocol is shown in Figure 5.1, and this illustrates the elements that make up a review. Throughout the remainder of this chapter we will guide you through these elements and take you through the exercise of constructing a review protocol for a systematic review of the question that you identified earlier.

Title

The title of your review will be drawn from the question that you are seeking to answer. This is no doubt self-evident, but some examples of review titles published by the Joanna Briggs Institute will illustrate the point.

Title	Author	Publication details
Association between pacifier use and breast-feeding, sudden infant death syndrome, infection and dental malocclusion	Callaghan et al.	2005, 3 (6)
Effectiveness of a pelvic floor muscle exercise program on urinary incontinence following childbirth	Haddow et al.	2005, 3 (5)
Effectiveness of topical skin care provided in aged care facilities	Hodgskinson & Nay	2005, 3 (4)
Knowledge retention from preoperative patient information	Stern & Lockwood	2005, 3 (3)
Effectiveness of primary conservative management for infants with obstetric brachila plexus palsy	Bialocerkowski et al.	2005, 3 (2)

The steps involved in the preparation of a review protocol will be apparent from the protocol illustrated above. In the following section we elaborate on what this entails.

In practice . . .

Think about young Harry with his asthma now. In addition to developing a protocol for the question that you generated in relation to your own practice, you may find it useful as you work through the following section to apply the information in developing a review protocol to suit the question that you identified earlier in relation to his case.

Background review

The initial step is to undertake a general evaluation of the literature to determine the scope and quantity of the primary research, to search for any existing reviews and to identify issues of importance. The background is an opportunity to provide context for the review question and a rationale for conducting the review. It is important that the review question and motivation for conducting the review is justified, clear and succinct. The background for a systematic review should include:

- A discussion of the review question itself and how it emerged.
- An assessment of the significance of the topic to health care.
- An overview of issues relevant to the review question.
- An overview of previous reviews of the review topic, or of topics related to it.
- A description of any controversies related to the review topic.

The background should describe the issue under review including the target population, interventions and outcomes that are documented in the literature. The background should be an overview of the main issues. It should provide sufficient detail to justify the conduct of the review and the choice of the various elements such as the interventions and outcomes. It is often as important to justify why elements are not included. In describing the background literature, value statements about effect of interventions should be avoided, for example: 'Use of acupuncture is effective in increasing smoking cessation rates in hospitalised consumers.' This is what the review will determine. If this type of statement is made, it should be clear that it is not the reviewer's conclusion but that of a third party, such as: 'Smith indicates that acupuncture is effective in increasing smoking cessation rates in hospitalised consumers.'

Existing research results may be conflicting, variations in current practice may be identified or potential gaps in the body of research may be motivating factors. The background should provide a clear and logical progression to your review question.

Objectives

As with any research, it is important to have a clear question, and the objective(s) of the review will flow from this question. The protocol should state in detail the questions or hypotheses that will be pursued in the review.

The articulation of objectives for the review can best be illustrated by example. For instance, in a review entitled *The effectiveness of mechanical compression devices in attaining hemostasis after removal of a femoral sheath following femoral artery cannulation for cardiac interventional procedures: a systematic review* (Jones, 2000), the objective was stated in the following way:

> The main objective of this review was to present the best available information on the effectiveness of mechanical compression devices in achieving hemostasis after removal of the femoral sheath from patients after cardiac interventions.
>
> The specific null hypothesis (H_0) tested was: there is no difference in the effectiveness of mechanical compression devices in attaining haemostasis after femoral sheath removal as compared with manual compression or other compression techniques.
>
> In addition to examining the efficacy of mechanical devices, another objective was to review patient tolerability of mechanical compression devices after femoral sheath removal.

A second example of the objectives for a review can be seen in the review entitled *Knowledge retention from pre-operative patient information: a systematic review* (Hodgkinson et al., 2000). Here the objective was stated as follows:

> The objective of this review was to present the best available evidence related to knowledge retention and/or correct performance of post-operative activities following pre-operative patient education.

The examples provide some indication of the approach to be adopted in spelling out the objectives of your review.

Inclusion criteria

The protocol must describe the criteria that will be used to select the literature. It is important to be precise in defining the inclusion criteria as the reader of the review report needs to know the focus and limitations of the review. Specifically, in developing inclusion criteria, it is important to address:

- The types of studies to be included (for example, randomised controlled trials, pseudo-randomised controlled trials; or interpretive studies).
- The intervention, activity or phenomenon (for example, pharmaceutical and non-pharmaceutical interventions for smoking cessation).
- The outcome (for example, smoking cessation, smoking reduction).
- The specific study populations (for example, adult males aged 18 years and over who have been smoking for at least five years).
- Language of publication (for example, English only; or English, German, Spanish and Japanese).
- The time period (for example, study reports published or made available 1999–2005).

Here again, some examples of inclusion criteria from published reviews may offer some guidance. The following inclusion criteria have been reproduced with permission from Stern and Lockwood (2005), from their review entitled *Knowledge retention from preoperative patient information*. The inclusion criteria were articulated as:

Types of participants
This review considered all studies that included adults in a hospital setting, either as inpatients or same-day surgical patients, who received some form of instruction before an operative procedure.

Types of intervention
Interventions of interest were those related to the evaluation of pre-operative patient education, instruction or teaching, and included assessment of the effectiveness of different:

(1) presentations:
- written information
- audio-visual aids
- computer-assisted instruction
- learning packages

(2) structures:
- group or individual teaching
- structured or unstructured programmes

(3) deliveries:
- pre-admission or post-admission

Types of outcome measure
The primary outcomes of interest were those associated with the understanding of the information related to the operative or post-operative period that were provided in the intervention and included:

(1) increased knowledge
(2) ability to perform post-operative activities
(3) time taken to teach skills

Types of studies
This review considered randomised controlled trials (RCTs) that evaluated some form of pre-operative patient education to enable the identification of current best evidence regarding providing patients with pre-operative instruction to increase their understanding and knowledge. All studies were categorised according to the NHMRC levels of evidence.

Stern and Lockwood clearly indicate the inclusion criteria for their review and this facilitates the replicability of the review.

Building your protocol: inclusion criteria

Now that you have developed your question, your title and your objectives, you should be in a position to stipulate your inclusion criteria.

Again, you may find it useful to look at the inclusion criteria in some other published reviews to familiarise yourself with the requirements for this element of the protocol.

Search strategy

The importance of developing a thorough search strategy cannot be stressed enough. A poorly structured search strategy can severely diminish the quality of the review, should it not identify research papers pertinent to your review question. The protocol should provide a detailed strategy that will be used to identify all relevant literature within an agreed time frame. This should include databases and bibliographies that will be searched, and the search terms that will be used.

Haddow et al. (2005) summarised their research strategy in the following way:

'All major electronic sources of information relevant to the topic (e.g. PubMed, CINAHL and the Cochrane Library) were searched to identify published and unpublished studies and previous work in the field. Printed journals were hand-searched and reference lists checked for potentially useful research. The review included any studies undertaken between 1981 and 2003. The search did not attempt to locate unpublished research before 1991.'

However, their full account of their search strategy was significantly more comprehensive and is reproduced with permission as follows:

Search strategy
To identify all relevant studies for the review, the search strategy included searches of:

• indexes of periodical articles (e.g. CINAHL, MEDLINE/PubMed, Current Contents, Science Direct);

- indexes of reports, theses and conference papers (e.g. Dissertation Abstracts, Conference Papers Index, National Research Register – UK);
- major sources of evidence-based practice information (e.g. Cochrane Collaboration, NHS Centre for Research and Dissemination, Agency for Healthcare Research Quality and clinical trials databases); and
- websites of nursing and midwifery organisations and other relevant agencies (e.g. MIRIAD – a database of midwifery resources, International Continence Foundation, Society of Urologic Nurses).

Individual strategies were developed for each source searched, adopting the different terminology of index thesauri and/or using the natural language terms of the topic. These strategies were undertaken because it has been established that difficulties can arise when using MeSH terms only to locate clinical trials. The main terms and search strategies used to located studies are listed in Appendix I.

In addition, journals were hand-searched, either online or in hard copy form, and search alerts for the topic were established to ensure that relevant papers were identified as they were published. To ensure that all recently published papers had been located, the most relevant journals were individually searched for the publication years of 2001 and 2002 at least. Most of this hand-searching was carried out over a longer publication period. For a list of all the major sources searched and journals included in the search alerts see Appendix II. The reference lists of relevant papers and research studies were examined for potentially useful links to research not previously located.

The importance of contacting experts in the field to ensure all relevant studies are located has been reported. In this review contact was made with experts who had been involved in systematic reviews about related topics and authors of highly relevant studies to the review.

All relevant studies with an English language abstract were located for assessment against the inclusion criteria.

This demonstrates the level of specificity required in documenting a search strategy. The importance of the search strategy to the quality of the review has prompted us to provide more practical assistance later in this chapter.

Building your protocol: search strategy

Remember, your search strategy needs to be structured and detailed. Think back to your question, objectives and inclusion criteria. These should provide you with a solid guide as to the type of information you are searching for. From here, you will need to decide which databases will be the most appropriate and the specific strategies you plan to utilise for each database.

Assessment criteria

It is important to assess the quality of the research to minimise the risk of an inconclusive review resulting from excessive variation in the quality of the studies. The protocol must therefore describe how the validity of primary studies will be assessed and any exclusion criteria based on quality considerations.

> **Building your protocol: assessment criteria**
>
> Locate a number of systematic reviews from different sources that address diverse topics and methods, and consider the way they approach the issue of assessing the quality of the studies included. Note any checklists that are used. Having done this, prepare assessment criteria for your review.

Data extraction

It is necessary to extract data from the primary research regarding the participants, the intervention, the outcome measures and the results. Accurate and consistent data extraction is critically important and often data extraction forms are utilised to achieve this. Examples of sheets developed for this purpose should be included as part of the protocol.

> **Building your protocol: data extraction tools**
>
> Locate a number of systematic reviews from different sources that address diverse topics and methods, and consider the way they approach the issue of extracting data from the studies included. Note any tools that are used. Having done this, prepare (or adapt) a data extraction tool for your review.

Data synthesis

It is important to combine the literature in an appropriate manner when producing a report. Statistical analysis (meta-analysis) or textual analysis (meta-synthesis) may or may not be used and will depend on the nature and quality of studies included in the review. While it may not be possible to state exactly what analysis will be undertaken, the general approach should be included in the protocol.

> **Learning activity**
>
> **Data synthesis**
> If you are unfamiliar with the concept of data synthesis, you may find it extremely useful to locate a number of systematic reviews from different sources that address diverse topics and methods, and examine the way they analyse the data from the studies included.

This completes the process of preparing the protocol for your systematic review. You will no doubt have realised the fundamental importance of the protocol to the quality of the review. The investment of time and energy in getting the protocol right is the best guarantee of a positive outcome. This point will be further discussed.

Learning activity

Think again about the question you developed earlier. Having read about the criteria for a review protocol, how successful do you think your question would be as a systematic review question? Using the information you now possess, attempt to revise your question and write your own systematic review protocol.

The importance of systematic reviews of evidence

The assumption of evidence-based practice is that there are things we need to know in order to conduct our practice professionally but there are substantial gaps in the knowledge available to us. Systematic reviews aim to expose the gaps in specific areas and provide pointers to the kinds of questions for which we need to find answers.

Sackett et al. (1997) argue that almost every time a medical practitioner encounters a patient they will require new information about some aspect of the patient's diagnosis, prognosis or management. This is no less true for other health professionals. The researchers note that there will be times when the question will be self-evident or the information will be readily accessible. This is increasingly the case as sophisticated information technology gets nearer and nearer to the bedside. Even so, there will be many occasions when neither condition prevails and there will be a need to ask an answerable question and to locate the best available external evidence. This requires considerably more time and effort than most health professionals have at their disposal, and the result is that most of our information needs go unmet.

Asking answerable clinical questions is not as easy as it sounds, but it is a skill that can be learned. Sackett et al. (1997) offer some very useful advice in the context of evidence-based medicine and the effectiveness of interventions. These sources can be extended beyond questions of effectiveness, to consider the appropriateness and feasibility of practices:

The Source of Clinical Questions (adapted from Sackett et al., 1997)

Assessment	how to properly gather and interpret findings from the history, physical examination and care
Aetiology	how to identify causes for problems
Differential diagnosis	when considering the possible causes of a consumer's clinical problems, how to rank them by likelihood, seriousness and treatability
Diagnostic tests	how to select and interpret diagnostic tests, in order to confirm or exclude a diagnosis, based on consideration of their precision, accuracy, acceptability, expense, safety, etc.
Prognosis	how to gauge the consumer's likely clinical course and anticipate likely problems associated with the particular disease and social context of the person

Therapy	how to select therapies that result in more benefits than harm for consumers and that are worth the effort and cost of using them
Prevention	how to reduce the chance of ill health by identifying and modifying risk factors, and how to detect early problems by screening and consumer education
Feasibility	how practical it is to implement a practice within a given clinical setting, culture or country
Appropriateness	how to understand the social context within which practice takes place
Meaningfulness	how to understand the experience of a given treatment, practice or intervention
Self-improvement	how to keep up to date, improve your clinical skills and run a better, more efficient clinical service

Although health professionals often want to answer very broad questions, generally speaking, the narrower a question is, the easier it is to conduct the review and the more useful the final product will be. If the reviewers are interested in finding out the most effective, appropriate and feasible way of improving the quality of life of people with emphysema, it is desirable to conduct a series of reviews based on specific, focused questions rather than a broad, all-encompassing review that includes different populations, interventions and outcomes.

Systematic reviews of evidence are of significant importance when determining the best available evidence for practice. One of the most important components of this process is to have a solid protocol and search strategy in order to be able to find relevant information and produce *meaningful* information upon which to base practice.

Decision toolkit

Decision	Tools	Evaluation
Where to search for the information you need to provide quality care and information to Harry and his parents	Search strategy Reliable databases containing research evidence	Did you find adequate information to begin the process of establishing the best available evidence for Harry and his parents?

Finding the evidence

Once the question, issue or problem is identified from the field, the next step is finding the evidence. In order to do this it is necessary to have knowledge of techniques used to unearth the evidence and make it available. Although systematic reviews and practice guidelines are designed to save practitioners time by presenting condensed information, it is important that these summaries of information are open to assessment, and this can only be ensured by accessing the process used in the review. Just as research (whether published or unpublished) can vary in quality, so can a search for the evidence.

The search strategy should be clearly described in the review protocol. Determining rigorous procedures for the search before commencing the review reduces the risks of error and bias. The first step in any search strategy is defining preliminary search terms or keywords and then using these to search appropriate electronic databases. This preliminary search enables the reviewers to identify other keywords and to modify them according to the thesaurus used in each data base. Databases most frequently used are:

- CINAHL
- PsycINFO
- Current Contents
- Cochrane Library
- DARE
- Health Technology Assessment Database

- AustRom
- MEDLINE
- Science Citation Index
- Embase
- Dissertation abstracts

CINAHL

The Cumulative Index to Nursing & Allied Health (CINAHL) database provides authoritative coverage of the literature related to nursing and allied health. In total, more than 1200 journals are regularly indexed; online abstracts are available for more than 800 of these titles.

PsycINFO

This database contains records of research in psychology and related behavioural and social sciences research from 1967 onwards.

Current Contents

This is an index of journal articles, reviews, meeting abstracts, editorials, and suchlike, and covers more than 7500 international journals of all disciplines, bibliographic information, including English-language author abstracts for approximately 85% of articles and reviews in the science editions.

The Cochrane Database of Systematic Reviews

The Cochrane Library contains the full text of regularly updated systematic reviews of the effects of health care carried out by the Cochrane Collaboration and protocols for reviews currently in preparation.

DARE

The Database of Abstracts of Reviews of Effectiveness (DARE) contains appraisals of systematic reviews not published in the Cochrane Database of

Systematic Reviews. Regular searching of bibliographic databases, hand-searching of key major medical journals and scanning grey literature identifies these reviews.

(Note: Grey literature is defined as being: 'That which is produced on all levels of government, academics, business and industry in print and electronic formats, but which is not controlled by commercial publishers.' (*GL '99*, 1999).

Health Technology Assessment Database

This database contains abstracts of completed technology assessments and ongoing projects conducted by members of the International Network of Agencies for Health Technology Assessment and other health technology agencies.

AustRom

AustRom includes 13 Australian databases, mostly bibliographic, including indexes to journals, books, newspaper articles, reports, theses and manuscripts, conference proceedings and audio-visual material. Subjects covered include law, criminology, education, architecture, sport, leisure, recreation, psychology, economics and health issues relating particularly to Australia.

Medline

Medline is widely recognised as the premier source for bibliographic and abstract coverage of biomedical literature. It contains more than 9.5 million records from more than 3900 journals. Abstracts are included for about 67% of the records.

Science Citation Index

The Science Citation Index (SCI®) provides access to current and retrospective bibliographic information, author abstracts, and cited references found in 3700 of the world's leading scholarly science and technical journals covering more than 100 disciplines.

Embase

Embase is a comprehensive pharmacological and biomedical database renowned for extensive indexing of drug information from 4550 journals published in 70 countries. It is one of the most current biomedical databases available. This database contains records of biomedical literature from 1974 onwards.

Dissertation abstracts

Dissertation Abstracts Online is a definitive subject, title, and author guide to virtually every American dissertation accepted at an accredited institution since

1861. Selected Masters theses have been included since 1962. In addition, since 1988 the database includes citations for dissertations from 50 British universities that have been collected by and filmed at The British Document Supply Centre. Beginning with DAIC Volume 49, Number 2 (Spring 1988), citations and abstracts from Section C, Worldwide Dissertations (formerly European Dissertations), have been included in the file. Abstracts are included for doctoral records from July 1980 (Dissertation Abstracts International, Volume 41, Number 1) to the present. Abstracts are included for Masters theses from Spring 1988 (Masters Abstracts, Volume 26, Number 1) to the present.

The world wide web

The internet may be a useful source of information regarding research that is in progress or yet to be formally published. However,searching the internet is a complex and time-consuming process, and while there are strategies to deal with the phenomenal amount of information available, it is not recommended unless deemed absolutely essential.

Searching

Because searching electronic databases is complex and requires a great deal of skill, it is important to work closely with a librarian when deciding which databases to search and what search terms to use in each of these. A number of potential problems can be avoided if a skilled librarian is involved. For example, differences in spelling conventions such as 'randomised' versus 'randomized' and 'paediatric' versus 'pediatric' can be overcome by using the thesaurus of specific databases. The same applies when different terms are used in different countries, such as the terms mucositis and stomatitis. There are also variations in controlled vocabulary between databases. MEDLINE, for example, uses the term cerebrovascular accident whereas cerebral vascular accident is used in CINAHL. Thus, in doing the search, it is important to utilise the aids available in databases.

Truncation is an aid in some databases that can be used to search for a number of words with the same stem. In some databases, if an asterisk is inserted at the end of such a word (for example restrain*) then the search will include words that contain that stem (such as restraint, restrained, restraining, etc.). Another useful aid is that of the 'wild card'. A wild card can be inserted in the place of a letter to pick up words that have different spellings. In some databases, the wild card is used by inserting a question mark (for example, randomi?ed) and any word with that spelling will be searched for (such as randomised and randomized).

Most reputable databases have a thesaurus or controlled vocabulary, which is a list of headings used to standardise the indexing in the database; it is important to use this when conducting searches. It is also useful if you want to narrow or broaden your search to use an aid called Boolean operators. This aid is used by inserting such terms as 'and' 'near' or 'not'.

It is also useful to be aware of the fact that the same research article may appear in more than one database, so it is important to ensure that you have an adequate system for managing the citations at this preliminary stage. Programs such as Endnote, Procite or Reference Manager may be useful, and some have the capacity to link into other programs such as Microsoft Word in order to produce reference lists for systematic review reports. Much of the new software being developed to assist with the systematic review process includes facilities to enable linking to such programs for the management of references.

Hand-searching

Not all journals are referenced in the electronic databases, and many other sources of evidence, such as conference papers and unpublished work, will be lost to the review if it is limited to only electronic searches. A comprehensive review therefore also includes manual searching of journals and the reference lists of articles and abstracts retrieved.

The logistics of a search

In developing a search strategy, and then following that strategy, the logistics need to be well thought through. It is useful to be clear about what databases and resources are going to be searched, as not all databases are accessible to reviewers and only those that can reasonably be utilised should be included.

Who will do the search?

Doing a comprehensive search is time-consuming, laborious and requires a degree of commitment. Someone who has the time, skill and commitment needs to be identified to do this, and a second reviewer with similar characteristics is also required.

What help will be available from librarians?

Although librarians may not be well versed in the substantive area of the review question, they are highly skilled in electronic searching and in the retrieval of papers. Conducting a search without the help of a librarian is not recommended! A search for articles related to smoking cessation may focus on systematic reviews evaluating the effectiveness or efficacy of interventions/strategies relating to smoking cessation in the hospitalised consumer. In the absence of this type of systematic review, those that evaluate interventions and programmes that may readily be applied to the hospitalised consumer may also be considered. In such an instance, the search would focus on accessing databases recognised as having a primary focus on health care outcomes by preparing and/or maintaining systematic reviews or clinical practice guidelines on the effects of health care interventions. Databases such as the Cochrane Collaboration Library, the Database of Abstracts of Reviews of Effectiveness (DARE), Health Services/Technology Assessment Text (HSTAT), Centers for Disease Control and Prevention (CDC), the Centre for Reviews and Dissemination (CRD), or the Joanna Briggs Institute (JBI) would be appropriate for this situation.

An example of a search strategy for acupuncture for smoking cessation may include terms such as:

- (smok* OR tobacco AND cessation)
- AND (acupuncture OR acupressure OR transcranial OR transcutaneous OR electrical stimulation OR electrostimulation OR electro?acupuncture OR neuro?electric therapy OR laser therapy)
- Limit to years 1990 to 2005
- RCT search strategy

Learning activity

Again, go back to your review protocol. Choose **one** database appropriate to your review topic and attempt to perform a search. Remember to be aware of language differences and to utilise the relevant limits for your search. This is a useful exercise that will help you to get a feel for the variations in research reports that are generated by a database search. From your search, select several articles for retrieval that you believe to be relevant to your review question for use in the next chapter.

Study selection

This search strategy may identify an extraordinary numbers of articles. Some of these may be definitively linked to your objective, or may possess a vague connection to one or more of the search terms utilised but be of no relevance to your review.

Examples of potentially relevant studies:

White, A. R., Rampes, H., Ernst, E. 2002 Acupuncture for smoking cessation. [update of Cochrane Database Syst Rev. 2000;(2):CD000009; PMID: 10796466]. [Review] [49 refs] [Journal Article. Review] Cochrane Database of Systematic Reviews. (2):CD000009, 2002.

He, D., Medbo, J. I. Hostmark, A. T. Effect of acupuncture on smoking cessation or reduction: an 8-month and 5-year follow-up study. [Clinical Trial. Journal Article. Randomized Controlled Trial] Preventive Medicine. 33(5):364–72, 2001 Nov.

Examples of probably irrelevant studies:

Vachiramon, A., Wang, W. C. Vachiramon, T. The use of acupuncture in implant dentistry. [Review] [66 refs] [Journal Article. Review. Review, Tutorial] Implant Dentistry. 13(1):58–64, 2004 Mar.

Haustein, K. O., Krause, J., Haustein, H., Rasmussen, T. and Cort, N. Effects of cigarette smoking or nicotine replacement on cardiovascular risk factors and parameters of haemorheology. [Clinical Trial. Journal Article] Journal of Internal Medicine. 252(2):130–9, 2002 Aug.

It is important that when selecting research articles that you intend to retrieve, you aim to select only those studies that are relevant to your review question. The process or strategy you utilise to select studies must be transparent and reproducible, and should relate back to the inclusion and exclusion criteria that were set out in the protocol. For example, the study needs to have been published within the time frame stated in the protocol (i.e. between 1990 and 2005), the population needs to meet the criteria set in the protocol (i.e. adult smokers aged between 18 and 60 years) and interventions or phenomena need to be stated in the review question (acupuncture as a smoking cessation strategy).

This is an initial assessment that occurs following the search, which addresses whether or not the paper should be *retrieved*. The second assessment, that of critical appraisal, occurs when the paper has been retrieved and addresses whether or not the study should be *included in the review*. It is essential to use two assessors in both the selection of papers and critical appraisal processes to limit the risk of error.

Once an exhaustive search has been conducted, the resulting titles (and abstracts, if available) are assessed to establish whether they meet the eligibility criteria set out in the protocol. Those articles that do not meet the inclusion criteria are rejected, but bibliographical details are recorded in a table for inclusion in the systematic review report. Some reviewers do not include this in the report (for example, Cochrane Reviews do not do so) whereas others do (for example, Joanna Briggs Institute reviews do include them in an appendix). If there is uncertainty about the degree to which an article meets the inclusion criteria or if the criteria are clearly met, the full text of the article is retrieved. Two reviewers then independently assess all of the retrieved articles. If both reviewers agree to accept or reject an article, this occurs; if there is disagreement, the reviewers should confer and reach agreement.

Documenting the search

In order for another reviewer to be able to replicate the systematic review, the search process needs to be as transparent as possible. Documenting the search will not only allow others to duplicate the process followed, but will also allow readers to evaluate the rigour with which the search was conducted. Any reasons for changes in the strategy or other decisions made along the way should be noted.

Conclusion

The basis of evidence-based practice – the systematic review – has been described in this chapter. Significant progress has been made in recent years with regard to extending the scientific methodology and philosophies that underpin the systematic review process. A particular achievement has been the evolution of the concept of evidence along with the broadening nature of evidence to be included in systematic reviews and thereby utilised as evidence for the facilitation of practice change. However, this has brought with it challenges not only with regard to critical appraisal and synthesis, but also for the classification of evidence for recommendations. To some extent the issues surrounding the inclusion of other forms of research evidence in the systematic review process have been overcome. This being the case, the challenge becomes one of development, implementation and audit of clinical guidelines.

In practice . . .

In your professional career you may or may not find due cause to initiate the conduct of a systematic review of research evidence. Regardless of whether this becomes a part of your professional life or not, it is likely that at some point you will have cause to read a systematic review. Thus, it is important to understand why they are of significance, and to appreciate the components that constitute a good review.

The next time you are searching for information on a given practice or intervention, consider where you are looking for that information and what information you might find (or, just as importantly, what you might miss) if you do not search thoroughly. Consider also the impact that utilising the wrong type of information might have on practice. How might such a mistake have impacted on Harry and his parents? Searching without a comprehensive strategy may result not only in inaccurate reviews of literature, but in wide variation in practice.

Further reading and resources

If you are interested in learning more about the material addressed in this chapter, we would suggest the following:

Day, J. (2001) The quest for information: a guide to searching the Internet. *The Journal of Contemporary Dental Practice* **2** (4): 1–4.

Littleton, D., Marsalis, S. and Bliss, D. Z. (2004) Searching the literature by design. *Western Journal of Nursing Research* **26** (8): 891–908.

Lowe, H. J. and Barnett, O. (1994) Understanding and using the medical subject headings (MeSH) vocabulary to perform literature searches. *Journal of the American Medical Association* **271** (14): 1103–08.

Other useful resources for locating research and information for inclusion in systematic reviews include:

ARIF appraisals: www.bham.ac.uk/arif/enqscomp.htm

Health Services/Technology Assessment Text: http://text.nlm.nih.gov/

National Coordinating Centre for Health Technology Assessment: www.hta.nhsweb. nhs.uk/

NICE appraisals: www.nice.org.uk/

TRIP: www.tripdatabase.com

Chapter 6

Evidence Synthesis: Critical Appraisal, Data Extraction and the Synthesis of Findings

'Probably all of us are prejudiced and tend to focus on what we like to see. And, even worse, some tend to dismiss anything that does not suit their purpose.' – P. Knipschild

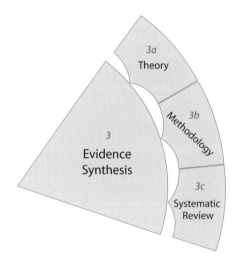

In Chapter 1 we explained the nature of evidence-based practice and the emergence and development of the evidence-based health care movement. In Chapter 2 we introduced the JBI Model of Evidence-Based Health Care and its components. In Chapter 3 we examined the nature of evidence and the various types of evidence that we consider to be useful for informing practice. In Chapter 4 we addressed the first of the substantive components of EBHC, which deals with the activity most fundamental to evidence-based practice, that is the generation of evidence. The basis of evidence-based practice is, of course, evidence. In Chapter 5 we moved on to the next component, that of the synthesis of evidence and began to take you through the process of the systematic review. In so doing, we dealt only with the first half of the systematic review, that is locating the evidence, leaving the second half – the appraisal and evaluation of the evidence – to Chapter 6. In this chapter, we will take you through the processes and issues associated with the synthesis of different forms of evidence, thus enabling you to complete a systematic review.

This chapter discusses:

- The appraisal of quantitative and qualitative evidence
- The extraction of quantitative and qualitative findings
- The synthesis of quantitative and qualitative findings
- Systems to manage the appraisal, extraction and synthesis of quantitative and qualitative evidence

---

In practice . . .

A high-powered executive who has been receiving treatment for stress and depression comes into your care. Sarah is working through some of her problems, one of which is her tendency to smoke at even higher levels during periods of extreme stress. She is well read and is keen to have a good understanding of all of the options available to her. You have identified significant literature regarding smoking cessation strategies. There are articles on everything from educational strategies to nicotine replacement therapy and acupuncture. You have selected studies for retrieval based on their title and abstract where available, but the results of the studies are variable and you now need to distinguish between studies that are of good quality and those that are not.

As you read through this chapter, keep in mind Sarah's situation. At various points you will be asked to think about how the content might relate to this case and whether it offers any solutions or strategies for assisting her.

Introduction

This chapter considers the appraisal, data extraction and data analysis or synthesis of different forms of evidence. As we have discussed in earlier chapters, determining what constitutes the 'best' evidence is dependent on the kind of question being addressed. If our interest was in the effects of a specific treatment on specific outcomes (for example, the effectiveness of dry dressings on the rate of wound healing), then the results of randomised controlled trials would represent the 'best' evidence. When such evidence is not available, the results of other quantitative studies that measure the relationship between the treatment and specified outcomes may be suitable sources of evidence. Similarly, if the focus of the question were on the prevalence or aetiology of a specific condition or phenomenon (for example, of pressure ulcers in nursing homes), the most appropriate evidence would be found in quantitative descriptive studies.

Questions that concern matters of feeling, meaningfulness or the feasibility of using a particular approach or treatment within a defined cultural or geographical context cannot usually be addressed through the conduct of a randomised trial as the nature of the question is essentially qualitative rather than some particular quantifiable entity. Data of this kind is usually generated through qualitative research or it is obtained from experts and therefore is textual in nature, rather than numerical.

The types of data generated from these different types of research require different strategies for critical appraisal, data extraction and data analysis or synthesis. It is these different strategies that will be examined during the course of this chapter, along with some practical tools to assist in the systematic review process.

In practice . . .

When you consider Sarah's situation, what kinds of research, and thus what kinds of data, are you likely to be most interested in accessing? In responding to this question, think back to the processes in previous chapters for arriving at these judgements.

Critical appraisal of evidence

All papers selected for inclusion in the systematic review (that is, those that meet the inclusion criteria described in the protocol) need to be subjected to rigorous appraisal by two critical appraisers. The purpose of appraisal is to include only those studies that are of high quality, and thus to exclude those of poor quality. Given that the systematic review aims to summarise the best available evidence through, where possible, pooling the results of sufficiently similar studies, it is important to note that the pooling of poor-quality evidence may lead to outcomes that are less than desirable for patients.

Critical appraisal is a difficult component of the systematic review process, and a good understanding of research design is required. The major aim of critical appraisal of any type of evidence is to establish the validity of the evidence for practice. Validity refers to the soundness of the evidence; in other words, it is about the degree to which we can accept the evidence as trustworthy and believable. Although there are well-accepted definitions of the term validity in relation to the measures or findings of quantitative research, when we assess the validity of evidence for health care practice these definitions are not the only ones that can be applied to evidence that arises out of other research designs or comes from the opinion of experts.

It is therefore important, when considering the critical appraisal of evidence for practice, to start from a broad understanding of the notion of validity before applying validity criteria to specific sources of evidence. No matter whether the evidence being appraised arises out of a randomised controlled trial (for example, a trial on the effects of aspirin on pain levels as measured by a visual analogue scale, where the results are analysed using statistical tests to identify statistical significance) or a qualitative study (for example a phenomenological study of people's experience of toothache where the words of the people themselves are the data and are analysed through the researcher's interpretation of the meanings people associate with toothache), the validity of the evidence still relates to the power it has to convince us that it is sound and supportable.

Thus, validity is essentially the quality of being logically valid. When the evidence arises out of research, validity is therefore inextricably linked with the rigour of the research process utilised. Criteria used to assess rigour differ according to the research traditions that underpin the research process reported. When evidence arises out of opinion, the validity or soundness of it, while still assessable by considering its logic and its ability to convince, is also dependent on the strength, force, or authority of the source and expression of the opinion – that quality of the opinion that renders it supportable.

In practice . . .

Taking into account Sarah's background and experience, do you think that she is more likely to be persuaded by data generated by RCT or by opinion evidence? Is this a relevant consideration in your deliberations on how best to assist her?

In practice . . .

By now it will be obvious to you that there are a variety of sources of data, and that the type of data will determine the kind of appraisal and the elements to be evaluated. You will recall that in Chapter 5 you conducted a search on the question around which you structured the protocol for your systematic review. You were asked to identify a number of articles for the purposes of this chapter. The best approach to familiarising yourself with the appraisal requirements for the different kinds of data is to take those articles and appraise them in accordance with the relevant checklists set out below for the particular kind of data as you work through the chapter. The first thing that you will need to do is to identify the kind of data each of the articles contains, for example whether it is quantitative or qualitative. You may also wish to ensure that you have articles that address different kinds of data to maximise the usefulness of this exercise.

Quantitative evidence

The validity of randomised or pseudo-randomised studies refers to the degree to which possible bias has been limited (Moher et al., 1995). Bias refers to any influence that may distort the results of a study. Relying on the results of RCTs with variable validity and pooling these results may lead to a conclusion that is incorrect and thus mislead us to conclude that an activity or intervention is effective when it is not, or vice versa. Sources of bias in RCT designs include selection bias, performance bias, attrition bias and detection bias.

Selection bias usually arises out of an inadequate randomisation of subjects. There are strategies that can be used to minimise the chance of bias (e.g. blinding until treatment allocation). Blinding in this context means ensuring that neither the researchers nor the subjects are aware of who is allocated to the control group or the experimental group. Randomisation should ensure that every participant has an equal chance of being in any of the study groups, and appraisers therefore need to establish how well this was achieved.

Randomisation of participants is of vital importance in a clinical trial. This prevents both the participants and the researchers from influencing the outcomes of the research. It is best achieved by an individual who is not directly linked to the study or by using a system whereby randomisation of participants cannot be in any way manipulated, such as blinding or allocation concealment.

When critically appraising a randomised controlled trial, there are a number of indicators as to whether or not true randomisation has occurred. For example, the presence of any of the following strategies in the design of the RCT is intended to achieve randomisation:

• Centralised or pharmacy-controlled allocation
• Pre-numbered or coded containers
• On-site computer system
• Sequentially numbered, opaque envelopes

Performance bias arises when there are differences in care received other than treatment. Performance bias is avoided by the concealment of the treatment group. It is essential that performance bias is limited in order to ensure that the study participants are protected against unintended differences in care and placebo effects. Again, this may be achieved through blinding both participants and carers to prevent 'contamination' or 'co-intervention' that may affect study results.

Attrition bias relates to differences in terms of losses of subjects between groups. It is important that all differences between study groups are reported. Losses to a study include things such as participants who withdraw or drop out or deviate from the original protocol in some way. Losses to follow-up should be reported, but this is sometimes difficult to assess.

Detection bias relates to differences that may occur when assessing the outcomes of study groups. Again, blinding is an important factor to consider when examining detection bias.

The same sources of bias are relevant in appraising descriptive studies but, because these types of studies are less able to address questions of cause and effect than the RCT, the sources of bias are interpreted differently in the appraisal process. In the case of case control studies, selection bias is minimised by identifying and dealing with potential confounding factors. In cohort studies, which are described later in this chapter, the degree to which the study sample is representative of the population is central to assessing validity.

There is disagreement internationally on the most appropriate way of carrying out the appraisal of RCTs, case control and cohort studies. These disagreements largely concern the number of appraisers required and whether or not (if there are two or more appraisers) the process should be carried out independently by each of the reviewers, what should occur if reviewers disagree, and what degree of expertise in research methods is necessary in reviewers. Notwithstanding the lack of consensus in this area, there is growing acceptance (as evidenced by the approaches adopted by many systematic review groups such as the Joanna Briggs Institute, the NHS Centre for Reviews and Dissemination and the Scottish Intercollegiate Guidelines Network) of the need for papers to be appraised independently by two reviewers, and for these reviewers to confer and reach agreement. There is also increasing allegiance to the view that reviewers should have previous training in the critical appraisal process and experience and training in research design.

Criteria for the appraisal of studies vary from centre to centre and it is generally accepted that criteria may be developed specifically for each review. Reviewers often design an appraisal sheet and pilot the criteria on a small number of papers to establish that the criteria are appropriate and that they discriminate between papers with obvious low or high risk bias. Other reviewers suggest, however, that as the aim is to appraise the degree to which bias has been limited, the criteria should be common to all studies of the same design.

Critical appraisal of randomised controlled trials and quasi experimental studies

The randomised controlled trial has long been considered the 'gold standard' for evidence of effectiveness. However, these types of studies still present limitations and there is the possibility that errors may arise as a result of bias or chance. There are several criteria that should be considered when undertaking critical appraisal of randomised controlled trials and quasi-experimental studies.

In our smoking cessation example, a randomised controlled trial may have been conducted to examine the effectiveness of exercise counselling to aid in smoking cessation. The aim of the study would be to examine whether exercise counselling increases smoking abstinence, and reduces tobacco withdrawal and gains in weight and body fat.

- It is important to first establish whether the patients were **randomised to study groups**. The method of allocation should be described in sufficient detail in the report to enable the appraiser to be confident that it was without bias. It should be noted that in some cases full randomisation might be either not feasible or inappropriate for the intervention of interest.

  The report may state that on attendance at their first treatment session individual smokers were assigned to either the exercise or the control condition, using a computer-generated list of random numbers. This would indicate that the allocation method occurred randomly and without bias.

- It should be clear to the appraiser whether **allocation to treatment groups was concealed from the allocator**. Other than the intervention(s), the participants should be treated the same. There should be no evidence of additional treatments given to one group in comparison to another.

  The report may state that exercise counselling was provided to the intervention groups. In all other aspects of smoking cessation support they were treated just the same as the control group. This would suggest that both groups were treated in the same way except for the intervention being evaluated.

- The groups included in the study should have been **comparable at entry**. There should be no measurable difference in the characteristics of the different treatment groups.

  The report may state that men and women aged 18 to 65 years, who had been smoking at least ten cigarettes a day for at least three years, were motivated to stop smoking and had not engaged in moderate daily exercise were recruited.

- The **outcomes should have been measured in the same manner for all participants**. It should be evident that those assessing outcomes were blinded to the treatment allocation. That is, they were not aware of whether the patient was allocated to the treatment group or the control group. It should also be clear that the outcomes were measured in a reliable manner.

  The report may state that in interviews conducted by a researcher who was unaware of the interviewee's group allocation, a structured interview schedule was followed to elicit data on the number of cigarettes smoked per day and the smoking patterns of the interviewee.

- The **statistical analysis used should have been appropriate for the data presented and the dropout rate not significant**. Generally a dropout rate of 5% or less is considered inconsequential and a rate of 20% or greater is considered as seriously impacting on the validity of the study.

  The report may state that 35% of subjects who entered the study withdrew and that all of these were followed up to establish the reasons for dropping out of the study and to elicit data on smoking frequency and patterns. (Data collected from those who dropped out may also be presented.) The report may also describe the statistical tests used to analyse data and justify their use.

- The rate of patient follow-up should be reported as adequate. **At least 80% of patients should have been followed up.**

Critically appraising cohort studies

Cohort studies examine a particular group of individuals over a designated period of time. As with critical appraisal of any research paper, there are study design features that are pivotal when undertaking critical appraisal of cohort studies.

In our smoking cessation example, a cohort study might be a prospective study of household smoking bans and subsequent cessation-related behaviour. The aim of the study would be to assess the degree to which smokers living with a full household ban on smoking change their cessation-related behaviour.

- It is essential that the choice of study method is appropriate. Usual types of studies include cohort/survival studies.

  The report may state that a prospective cohort study was conducted, utilising baseline and follow-up surveys.

- The population should be appropriate and sufficiently broad in representation.

  The report may state that in year one a telephone survey was conducted with 6199 adult, English-speaking members of the community, and in year two a follow-up survey was conducted with 1604 individuals who were smokers or living in a household with at least one smoker in the initial survey.

- The control group used was appropriate. If a comparison group is receiving an alternative therapy, consider whether this group is otherwise sufficiently similar.

The report may state that there were differences in the demographic characteristics of those who ceased smoking and those who didn't, and that the data were adjusted for the identified difference.

- All possible effect explanations are acknowledged. The study should address any additional factors that may impact on the outcomes.

  The report may state that factors such as differences in the age and socio-economic status of subjects between groups may have given rise to the findings. In such a case, there should be an explanation of how the results were adjusted for in the analysis to address the possible impact of the differences.

- The outcomes are objectively measured. It is important that those measuring the outcome are, where possible, blinded to the patients' clinical characteristics.

  The report may clearly define the outcome so that it is objective and not open to misinterpretation; for example, smoking cessation behaviour may be defined as number of cigarettes smoked or time between cigarettes.

- The duration of follow-up was adequate. The follow-up should be for a period that would allow the outcomes to occur.

  The report may state that subjects were followed up for a period that was long enough to detect the sustainability of smoking cessation. (It is important to remember that outcomes such as this can take a long time to establish. If follow-up is incomplete, the validity of the study may be severely threatened.)

- The effect was sufficiently long term. The effect or outcome measures should not be inconsequential.

  The report may state that smoking cessation (the outcome of interest in this study) was highly likely in homes with a total smoking ban and that the outcome is sustained for over a year.

- The dropout rate was not significant. Generally a dropout rate of 5% or less is considered inconsequential and a rate of 20% or greater is considered as seriously impacting on the validity of the study.

  The report may state that participants were followed up for a period of two years (i.e. follow-up lasted until a reasonable assessment could be made of the effects of the smoking ban on smoking cessation). If follow-up is short, it may be that study patients who cease smoking, do so for only a brief period and then recommence.

- The rate of patient follow-up was adequate. At least 80% of patients should have been followed up.

  The report may state that 85% of patients were followed up for a period of two years. The more subjects who are unavailable for follow-up, the less accurate the estimate of the effects of smoking bans on smoking cessation will be.

Critically appraising case control studies

Case control studies are often utilised to investigate the cause of a disease or the adverse effects of a treatment or intervention. However, they are also prone to bias, which makes critical appraisal a necessity. There are several criteria that should be considered when undertaking critical appraisal of case control studies.

In our smoking cessation example, a case control study may seek to examine the association between folate intake and risk of lung cancer in former smokers.

- Confounding factors should be identified and strategies to deal with them stated.

  The report may state that the proportion of cases with a history of asthma was higher in the folate intake cases than in the non-folate intake cases and that strategies to address the possible effect that this may have had on the occurrence of lung cancer were employed.

- There should be a statement regarding whether bias has been minimised in relation to selection of cases and of controls.

  The report may state that the investigators attempted to minimise bias by assembling people with a sole diagnosis of lung cancer as the cases and excluded patients with multiple cancers that included lung cancer; and included only patients who were receiving the same chemotherapy/radiotherapy.

- It should be clear to the appraiser that outcomes were assessed using objective criteria.

  The report may state that radiologically confirmed lung cancer was the outcome of interest.

- The outcomes of people who withdrew should be described and included in the analysis.

  The report may state that all withdrawn cases were followed up for an extended period and that a diagnosis/non-diagnosis of lung cancer occurring in withdrawn cases is included in the results.

- It should be evident that those outcomes were measured in a reliable way and that an appropriate statistical analysis was used.

Issues to be considered when appraising quantitative evidence

A major problem in the critical appraisal of all quantitative studies is that it depends solely on the detail of the paper, and appraisal is therefore just as much about the quality of the reporting as it is about the quality of the study itself.

Once the two appraisers have conferred and reached agreement on their rating, a decision is made on whether or not the study is of sufficient merit to be included in the review. This decision amounts to an evaluation of whether the study is sufficiently rigorous and the findings are sufficiently trustworthy to be included in the review. Some reviewers exclude any study that fails to meet one or more of the validity criteria, while others will identify 'critical criteria' that must be met and others set a minimum 'score' (e.g. six or more of ten criteria merit inclusion).

Qualitative evidence

Critically appraising interpretive and critical studies

As we have discussed previously, the major aim in critically appraising experimental or quantifiable data is to limit bias and thus establish the validity of a study. From a quantitative perspective, sources of bias include selection bias, performance bias and attrition bias, and validity is assessed by establishing the extent to which a study design and conduct addresses potential bias.

This focus on limiting bias to establish validity is antithetical to the philosophical foundations of qualitative approaches to inquiry. Emden and Sandelowski (1998) suggest that validity, in quantitative terms, measures those things that purport to render them generalisable. In social inquiry, however, they argue that validity is perceived in a different way as criteria of rigour for qualitative research.

There is much dissent in the literature on the appropriateness of establishing criteria to assess the validity of qualitative research. However, Pearson (2003) takes the view that a transparent approach to appraising qualitative research is central to its ongoing credibility, transferability and theoretical potential. Denzin and Lincoln (1994) concur with this and argue that there is a need for the development of a set of validity criteria sensitive to the nature of the qualitative research and its basis in subjectivity. Popay et al. (1998) are unequivocal in their assertion that the development of standards for assessing evidence from qualitative research is both possible and desirable, and set out the following as a guide to common standards:

- Evidence of responsiveness to social context and flexibility of design
- Evidence of theoretical or purposeful sampling
- Evidence of adequate description
- Evidence of data quality
- Evidence of theoretical and conceptual adequacy
- Potential for assessing typicality

There is a growing literature on the appraisal of qualitative studies and a large number of formats are available. Based on the literature and an extensive process of development and piloting, Pearson (2003) describes a general set of criteria for appraising the validity of interpretive and critical research.

In our smoking cessation example, a study may investigate the experiences of mental health clients as they relate to smoking behaviour, and the relationship of smoking behaviour to the course of their mental illness and its management, and to their attempts to quit smoking.

- It should be evident that there is congruity between the stated philosophical perspective and the research methodology. The report should clearly state the philosophical or theoretical premises upon which the study was based and the methodological approach adopted.

  The report may state that the study adopted an interpretive perspective and a survey methodology was followed. There is congruence between an interpretive view (focusing on knowledge arising out of studying what phenomena mean to individual groups) and surveys (an approach that focuses on asking standard questions to a defined study population).

- There is congruity between the research methodology and the research question or objectives. The study methodology should be appropriate for addressing the research question.

    The report may state that the research question was to seek understanding of the meaning of smoking in a group of people with mental illness and that a phenomenological approach was taken. Here there is congruity between the question and the methodology.

- There is congruity between the research methodology and the methods used to collect data. The data collection methods of the study should be appropriate to the chosen methodology.

    The report may state that the study pursued a phenomenological approach and data was collected through interviews. Here there is congruity between the methodology and data collection.

- There is congruity between the research methodology and the representation and analysis of data. The data should be analysed and represented in ways that correspond with the methodological position.

    The report may state that the study pursued a phenomenological approach to explore people's experience of smoking cessation by asking participants to describe their experiences of trying to quit. If the text generated from asking these questions is searched to establish the experience of smoking cessation for participants, and the experiences of all participants are included in the report findings, then there is congruity between the methodology and the representation and analysis of data.

- There is congruity between the research methodology and the interpretation of results. The results should be interpreted in ways that are reflective of the chosen methodology.

    The report may state that the study pursued a phenomenological approach to explore people's experience of attempts at smoking cessation and the results are used to inform practitioners about the differences in smoking patterns and needs for patients with mental illness. There is congruence between the methodology and this approach to interpretation.

- There is a statement locating the researcher culturally or theoretically. The beliefs and values of the researcher have the potential to influence the study, so it is important that these are addressed.

    The researcher plays a substantial role in the qualitative research process and it is important, in appraising evidence that is generated in this way, to know the researcher's cultural and theoretical orientation. A high-quality report will include a statement that clarifies this.

- The influence of the researcher on the research, and vice versa, is addressed.

    Any relationship the researcher has to an element of the research (i.e. participants or process) should be acknowledged and addressed.

- Participants, and their voices, should be adequately represented. Generally, reports of this nature should provide illustrations from the data to show the basis of their conclusions and to ensure that the participants are represented in the report.

   The report may provide illustrations from the data to show the basis of their conclusions and to ensure that participants are represented in the report, such as, 'When I am well, I can do without a smoke for ages. I can stop just like that! When I am unwell, I'll smoke my head off.'

- The research should be identifiable as ethical either according to current criteria or, for recent studies, where there is evidence of ethical approval by an appropriate body. This is usually identifiable as a statement regarding the ethical approval process.

   The report may include a statement indicating that ethical approval was sought from the appropriate institution such as, 'Ethical approval was gained from the medical centre committee on clinical investigation.'

- Conclusions drawn in the research should appear to flow from the analysis, or interpretation of the data. This criterion concerns the relationship between the findings reported and the views or words of study participants. In appraising a report it is important that the appraiser is satisfied that the conclusions that have been drawn by the research are based on the data collected.

   The report may state that findings suggest there may be differences in smoking patterns and needs according to the person's psychiatric diagnosis and that it would be worthwhile to take this into account when attempting to help people with mental illness to quit.

Issues to be considered when appraising interpretive and critical research evidence

Critical appraisal of qualitative work, much as with quantitative work, is largely dependent on the detail of the paper, and appraisal is therefore just as much about the quality of the reporting as it is about the quality of the study itself. Again, once the two appraisers have conferred and reached agreement on their rating, a decision is made on whether or not the study is of sufficient merit to be included in the review. This decision amounts to an evaluation of whether the study is sufficiently rigorous and the findings are sufficiently trustworthy to be included in the review. As with quantitative studies, some reviewers exclude any study that fails to meet one or more of the validity criteria while others will identify 'critical criteria' that must be met and others set a minimum 'score' (e.g. six or more out of ten criteria merit inclusion).

Critically appraising economic evaluation studies

Over the last decade interest in economic evaluation of health care interventions has escalated, with systematic reviews increasingly including economic evaluations to complement evidence related to clinical effectiveness. Studies that evaluate the economics of an intervention, activity or service attempt to compare different interventions, activities or services in terms of both the costs and the outcomes. There are a number of approaches to the economic evaluation of health care practices and the field is complex, largely understood only by experts in health economics. The dominant approaches in this field are:

- Cost minimisation studies
- Cost-benefit analyses
- Cost-effectiveness analyses
- Cost-utility analyses

Cost minimisation refers to studies of situations where there are two or more interventions or services that are known to achieve comparable outcomes and a cost analysis of the different interventions is conducted to identify the intervention of least cost. Cost-effectiveness analysis is carried out in situations where outcomes are not equivalent and often, in this approach, the differences in costs and actual outcomes (for example, wound healing rates) are analysed to elicit relationships between costs and relative effectiveness (for example, the costs per wound healed using moist dressings compared to costs using dry dressings). In cost-utility analysis (a form of cost-effectiveness analysis) the outcome is measured in quality life years (QALY), which is a measure of the changes in the years of survival of patients and their quality of life in terms of independence, presence of symptoms etc. In cost–benefit analysis the outcomes focused on are given a monetary value and the aim is to determine whether or not the costs outweigh the benefits or vice versa. Measures typically used in economic evaluations are actual costs, measures of effectiveness, incremental cost-effectiveness ratios and degrees of uncertainty.

Nixon et al. (2004) recognised the challenges faced by reviewers in collating, appraising and synthesising economic evidence to assist in decision-making about the costs of competing alternatives. Considerable gaps have been identified in the quality of reporting and methods applied to economic evaluations of health care interventions. They conclude that existing methods for summarising the results of economic evaluations within systematic reviews have some limitations for clinicians and policy makers because the methods must be interpreted using the textual and diagrammatic summaries normally provided. They propose that a hierarchical method provides an instant summary of findings in terms of effectiveness or benefit and in terms of cost.

When critically appraising economic evaluation reports, the same broad quality criteria can be applied to all approaches.

In our smoking cessation example, a study might conduct a cost-effectiveness analysis of a family-physician-delivered smoking cessation programme and compare the results to other smoking cessation interventions.

- Is there a well-defined question?
    Is it clear what interventions/programmes and outcomes will be examined in terms of cost effectiveness? Many economic studies are conducted in conjunction with clinical trials. The economic evaluation may relate to all or only part of the trial con-

ducted. The 'research question' stated in the paper often relates to the primary clinical trial and not the economic evaluation.

- Is there comprehensive description of alternatives?

  All interventions subject to the economic evaluation must be comprehensively described. Some interventions can be administered in a variety of ways that will impact on cost. Consider issues of duration and frequency of the intervention and mode of delivery, including level and type of practitioner. Consider if a 'do nothing' alternative is appropriate.

- Are all important and relevant costs and outcomes for each alternative identified?

  In delivering even a single simple intervention, there are a variety of costs incurred. These can be direct or indirect costs. An intervention may also result in benefit that reduces cost. An example of an 'avoided cost' is an intervention that reduces the rate of infection and subsequently reduces the cost of managing the infection. Consider costs to the health provider, the individual receiving the intervention and potentially also the individual's family.

- Are costs and outcomes measured accurately?

  A description should be given of how costs were derived. Any items included in the costings should have the 'price' or cost per unit reported separately from quantities used. This will assist in making judgements about the accuracy of measures. Consider the appropriateness of the physical units costed. Were they actual costs or estimates based on modelling? If costs were estimated, is the method logical?

- Are costs and outcomes valued credibly?

  The value of a cost or an outcome may vary depending on the perspective used to derive the value. In considering the outcome of pain, this may be valued in terms of the cost of analgesia (providers' perspective). For the patient, the emphasis is more likely to relate to the physical and emotional impact of pain.

- Are costs and outcomes adjusted for differential timing?

  Some interventions are ongoing and can incur costs into the future. Costs may be expected to change over time and therefore must be adjusted or 'discounted' to their value at the time of the intervention.

- Is there an incremental analysis of costs and consequences?

  In some cases it is appropriate to use the average cost of an intervention but in other cases the marginal (additional) cost of providing the intervention is more appropriate. The incremental cost is determined by establishing the difference between the marginal costs and consequences of the alternative interventions. If this approach is taken it should be justified.

- Were sensitivity analyses conducted to investigate uncertainty in estimates of cost or consequences?

  In some economic evaluations, certain costs and consequences are estimated on values that may vary over a range or have some degree of uncertainty. These elements in the evaluation are estimated using various assumptions. A sensitivity analysis is conducted to test the robustness of the result of the evaluation by varying these under-lying assumptions.

- Do study results include all issues of concern to users?
   This issue in part relates to perspective, and the interests of all stakeholders should be considered. There may be important ethical and cultural considerations.

- Are the results generalisable to the setting of interest in the review?
   Economic evaluations are conducted within a given context, taking into account a given population, health care setting, time and other elements that can impact on the generalisability of the results. In considering the clinical question that prompted the review of the economic evaluation, these elements should be considered in determining how widely the results can be used.

Critically appraising expert opinion

As we have discussed previously, the major aim in critically appraising expert opinion as it appears in publications and reports is to assess its validity as a source of guidance for practice when the results of rigorous inquiry on the question do not exist. Although research can be regarded as the most desirable approach to evidence generation, and thus the results of rigorous research can legitimately be seen to have a higher level of quality or validity than other sources of evidence, it is not unusual within the broad field of health care to find that expert opinion is the 'best available' evidence on a given topic.

Whether it is expressed by an individual, by a learned body, or by a group of experts in the form of a consensus guideline, expert opinion draws on the experience of practitioners. Thus, validity in this context relates to the soundness of opinion in terms of its logic and its ability to convince, the authority of the source and the quality of the opinion that renders it supportable. While expert opinion is rightly claimed to not be a product of 'good' science, it is empirically derived and mediated through the cognitive processes of practitioners who have typically been trained in scientific method. This is not to say that the superior quality of evidence derived from rigorous research is to be denied. However, in the absence of evidence derived from rigorous research, it is not appropriate to discount expert opinion as non-evidence.

Regarding expert opinion, viewing the words or text used to present it as data and reviewing this type of data within the systematic review process is not well recognised in the mainstream evidence-based health care movement, and (as we have discussed in earlier chapters) this is a source of criticism of evidence-based practice within the ranks of health care practitioners.

Pearson (2003) describes processes designed to examine text in documents, reports and consensus guidelines. The process seeks to locate the major themes in text that represents expert opinion. Approaches to critically appraise such nebulous and often conflicting data will always at best be tentative. This is not, however, a sufficient objection to rule out the use of a transparent process designed to identify the best available evidence for practice when results of research are not available. Appropriate sources of such evidence are therefore any text in which an informed opinion on the benefits or otherwise of an intervention or practice is manifested; that is, any statement in a particular medium such as a journal article, book, report or guideline that informs practice that emanates from a source that is regarded as authoritative by practitioners.

Establishing validity in this area is, then, something of a methodological and political minefield! McHoul and Grace (1993), in examining the analysis of discourse, cite Foucault's definition of discourse as 'historically specific, relatively well-bounded bodies of social knowledge' and describe processes that focus on examining the dominant messages that make up the opinion; analysing how these messages are constructed; identifying the credibility of the source of the opinion; establishing the motives that underlie these messages; and locating alternative messages that are given credence or, conversely, silenced. Validity in this context therefore relates to what is being said, the source and its credibility and logic; and consideration of the overt and covert motives at play.

There is much dissent in the literature on the appropriateness of referring to expert opinion as evidence, and there has been little work published on establishing criteria to assess the validity of text that does not emerge from a rigorous process of inquiry. We take the view that a transparent approach to appraising expert opinion is central to identifying the best available evidence for practice. This is not always easy to establish. However, there are some criteria that should be considered when undertaking critical appraisal of narrative, text and expert opinion papers.

In our smoking cessation example, an occasional review paper may have been published that addresses the promotion of smoking cessation in developing countries and proposes a framework for urgent public health interventions.

- In order to be able to assess an opinion, it is important that the source of the opinion is clearly identified.
  The text should clearly identify who the authors are.
- It should be possible to identify whether the source of the opinion has standing in the field of expertise.
  The author's qualifications, affiliations or professional standing should be identified.
- It should be possible to identify whether the interests of patients are the central focus of the opinion.
  Does the paper take a position that advantages a profession or a specific institution or body, rather than patients, clients, communities or health gain?
- The basis of the opinion in logic/experience should be clearly argued and explicit.
  The opinion should make sense, demonstrate an attempt to justify the stance it takes, and be the result of an analytical process that draws on experience or the literature.
- There should be reference to the extant literature/evidence.
  The authors should present evidence to support their arguments, and any incongruence should be addressed and justified.
- It should be clear whether or not peers support the opinion.
  The extent to which the opinion is supported or refuted by the current knowledge or practice base should be clear.

Learning activity

By now you should have found the appropriate checklists for the particular articles that you identified for appraisal. Regardless of the quality of the articles, we believe you will have found this to be an interesting exercise as it provides an opportunity to examine the process and see how the various criteria enable you to identify papers of various qualities. It may also have illustrated some of the complicating factors that can make sound critical appraisal such a time-consuming stage of the review process.

The limitations of critical appraisal

Critically appraising evidence is complex, time-consuming and characterised by an ongoing debate on how quality can best be determined across the broad spectrum of evidence types. Central to this debate are the reliance of appraisers on published reports and the lack of agreement on appropriate appraisal processes.

Many reports published in the refereed journals fail to provide sufficient detail to permit adequate appraisal. The emergence of evidence-based health care that incorporates critical appraisal has begun to have an influence on journals and authors in this regard, and there are signs that greater methodological detail is now present in a growing number of reports. However, inadequate reporting of research findings continues to be a common feature in all clinical fields and in relation to all research traditions.

As a result, even if a reported study may well have met the criteria set in evaluating validity, the report may not include information on, for example, the randomisation process used in an RCT or the relationship between the researcher and the participants in an action research study. Appraisers cannot assume that the study reported did meet the criteria if evidence for this is not explicit in the report. Some reviewers, in such a situation, contact the researchers involved to seek further information and this is generally appropriate. However, this is time-consuming and it is not unusual for reviewers to finds themselves in a position where the researchers cannot be located.

We will never reach total agreement on 'what counts as evidence' or on how evidence of all types can be appraised. There is a need for further research on criteria for assessing the validity of all types of evidence; improving standards for reporting study results; and empirical studies on the relationship between appraisal approaches and the validity of evidence.

The value of a research paper will depend on the relevance of the research objectives, the validity of the evidence and the sufficiency of the evidence provided to support claims made in the conclusion (Avis, 1994). Although there is no hard and fast set of criteria for making such judgements, a checklist of criteria can assist in identifying weaknesses. Critical appraisal is not intended as a stand-alone method for decision-making with regard to implementation of research results. Rather, its value lies in possessing the ability to be critical and sceptical of research reports and evidence represented in research papers and in utilising research as a means of questioning approaches to health care practices (for critical appraisal tools, see Appendix 2).

Critical appraisal of research evidence is one of the most difficult components of the systematic review process. The purpose of appraisal is to include only those studies that are of high quality and thus to exclude those of poor quality in order to produce *meaningful* information upon which to base practice that results in improved outcomes for patients.

Decision toolkit

Decision	Tools	Evaluation
How to assess the quality of the identified research evidence?	Choose the critical appraisal tool appropriate for the type of study you are assessing.	Were you able to assess the quality of the research and provide the best evidence to Sarah?

Data extraction

The data utilised in a systematic review are the results of individual studies, and they are collected with the aid of a data collection tool. Data is collected with the assistance of a tool in order to achieve a number of things. Data collection tools are used to ensure all of the relevant data is collected; to minimise the risk of transcription errors while data is collected; to allow the accuracy of data to be checked; and to serve as a record of the data collected.

Although actual data to be collected varies with each review, it always relates to the review question. This phase of the review may be complicated by factors such as incomplete reporting of study findings, the large range of outcomes commonly used to evaluate an intervention, and the different ways in which data is reported and presented.

Quantitative data extraction

Regardless of whether you utilise an established data extraction form or create and pilot your own, there are some key components of which you should be aware. It is important to collect information about the study references and reviewers, and about verification of study eligibility for the review. Then it is necessary to collect data related to the study characteristics such as the method, participants, interventions, outcome measures and results.

Quantitative methods include randomised controlled trials, experimental designs, quasi-experimental (pre/post test and post-test), and observational (correlational and descriptive). It is important when extracting information related to quantitative methods of research to be as specific as possible.

Reviewers will need to extract data related to the study population, the intervention, outcome measures and results. Characteristics of the populations studied may vary quite considerably and so it is important to collect information regarding such matters as age, gender, educational level, ethnicity and so on, as deemed relevant.

The exact form and delivery of the intervention should be detailed. An intervention is a planned change that has been made to the research environment by the researcher as part of the research project, and in quantitative research this information may take the form of routes of delivery, doses, timing, or length of treatment regimen. It is important to know as much as possible about the details of the intervention in order to be able to evaluate studies later and potentially combine the data collected.

Reporting of outcome measures can also vary considerably, meaning that reviewers will need to decide what information will best answer or inform the review question.

As the data for a systematic review is the results from individual studies, there are some difficulties that may arise when extracting data, such as:

- Different populations used
- Different outcome measures
- Different scales or measures used
- Interventions administered differently
- Reliability of data extraction (i.e. between reviewers)

However, there are some strategies you may wish to employ to minimise the risk of error when extracting data from quantitative studies. For example, you can:

- Utilise a data extraction form that is developed specifically for each review
- Pilot-test extraction form prior to commencement of review
- Train and assess data extractors
- Have two people extract data from each study
- Conduct the data extraction blind (i.e. without talking to your co-worker) prior to conferring

For those new to the systematic review process, it is recommended that they use an existing tool with established reliability.

In practice . . .

If any of the articles that you identified in your search are of a quantitative nature, you may wish to extract from them the relevant data using one of the data extraction tools illustrated above.

Qualitative data extraction

Just as with quantitative data extraction, qualitative data extraction involves transferring findings from the original paper using an approach agreed upon and standardised for the specific review. Thus, an agreed format is essential in order to minimise error, and to provide a historical record of decisions made about the data set for categorisation and synthesis. Again, regardless of whether you utilise an established data extraction form (of which, it should be noted, few exist for qualitative data) or create and pilot your own, there are some key components of which you should be aware.

Initial data extraction for qualitative studies varies little from that used for quantitative studies. It is important to collect information regarding the study references and reviewers, and about verification of study eligibility for the review. Then it is necessary to collect specific data related to the methodology, method, interventions, setting, geographical context, cultural context, participants, data analysis and authors' conclusions.

The methodology covers the theoretical underpinnings of the research. When extracting information regarding the study methodology it is important to include as much detail as possible. Below is a list of commonly used qualitative methodologies.

Action/description	Subjectivity (structures of consciousness)	Analytical
Ethnography	Phenomenology	Conceptual/analytical
Grounded theory	Ethnomethodology	Historical
Action research	Hermeneutic phenomenology	Discourse analysis
Case studies		Biographical/textual/narrative
Descriptive		Cultural/media analysis
Program evaluation		Deconstructive analysis

The method is the way in which the data is collected and a list of methods is provided below:

- Interview
- Media analysis
- Field notes
- Discourse analysis
- Observation
- Survey
- Questionnaire

It is important when extracting information about the method that you are as specific as possible. For example, if you are extracting data on a study that utilised interviews as its method, you need to specify whether the interview was open-ended, semi-structured, and conducted face-to-face or over the telephone.

As in quantitative research, an intervention is a planned change that has been made to the research environment by the researcher as part of the research project. There is not always an intervention in qualitative research, because much of this type of research is concerned with a particular phenomenon of interest.

The setting and geographical and cultural context are fairly self-explanatory. Here, you are extracting information related to the specific location of the research in terms of local environment (e.g. nursing home, acute care hospital, home), the country (Poland, United States, Australia, Thailand), and the cultural features in the study setting such as time period, ethnic groupings, age-specific groupings and socio-economic characteristics. Again, as with other data, when extracting data regarding cultural context it is important to be as specific as possible. This data should identify cultural features such as employment, lifestyle, ethnicity, age, gender, socio-economic class, location and time.

Information extracted regarding participants involved in the research should be related to inclusion and exclusion criteria of the research. It should also include, but not be limited to, descriptions of age, gender, number, participation rate, ethnicity, level of functionality and cultural background. Included here should be definitions of terms used to group people that may be ambiguous or unclear; for example, a carer is a personal care attendant.

Finally, you should collect data related to the data analysis techniques utilised in the research and the conclusions drawn from the analysis. Include here software programs that may have been used, contextual analysis, comparative analysis, thematic analysis, discourse analysis or content analysis. You may also wish to make comment at this stage about the overall quality of the paper. (For data extraction tools, see Appendix 3.)

Learning activity

Take the papers you have identified as being of good quality following critical appraisal and use the tools you now possess to extract the relevant information from those that are qualitative in nature.

Data analysis and synthesis

Whether discussing a quantitative combination of research results (commonly referred to as 'meta-analysis') or a qualitative combination of research results (commonly referred to as 'meta-synthesis'), we are essentially concerned with the pooling of results from 'like' studies. And regardless of the nature of the evidence being pooled, an open and explicit approach is required so that any comprehensive appraisal and synthesis of relevant studies may be critiqued and duplicated by others.

Meta-analysis and meta-synthesis are vitally important within the systematic review process and for evidence-based practice as they provide an opportunity to examine a larger data set than is generally achievable when conducting a single study.

When conducting data analysis there is a variety of information that can be reported in different ways. This includes what interventions or activities have been evaluated, the effectiveness/appropriateness/feasibility of the intervention or activity, what interventions may be effective, contradictory findings and conflicts, limitations of study methods, issues related to study quality, the use of inappropriate definitions, specific populations excluded from studies, and future research needs. These are all important issues to consider when you begin to conduct data analysis or synthesis.

Quantitative data analysis

When conducting a review of effectiveness, data is collected from individual studies and statistical methods can be used to analyse and summarise these data. If used appropriately, these methods provide a powerful tool for deriving meaningful conclusions from the data and help prevent errors in interpretation. Meta-analysis is useful when studies report different treatment effects or when studies are too small (insufficient power) to detect meaningful effects. Meta-analysis is also useful because of the simple fact that single studies rarely, if ever, provide definitive conclusions regarding the effectiveness of an intervention. Meta-analysis can be used if studies have the same population, use the same intervention administered in the same way, measure the same outcomes and are generally homogenous in nature. It is important, however, to note that meta-analysis of research data is not without limitations and its conduct does not guarantee that the results of a review are any more valid than those of a primary research study.

The methodologies developed by the Cochrane Collaboration for the meta-analysis of data from individual studies have remained significant since its inception.

Meta-analysis entails consideration of the following questions:

- What comparisons should be made?
- What study results should be used in each comparison?
- Are the results of studies similar within each comparison?
- What is the best summary of effect for each comparison?
- How reliable are those summaries?

Dichotomous data

Dichotomous data can be characterised when an individual is in one of two states. Such data can be summarised using odds ratio, risk ratios or risk difference.

Odds ratio: Odds ratio is the ratio of the odds of an event in the intervention group to the odds of an event in the control group. An odds ratio of one indicates no difference between comparison groups. For undesirable outcomes, an odds ratio of less than one indicates that the intervention was effective in reducing the risk of that outcome.

Relative risk: When we use the term 'relative risk', we are referring to the ratio of risk in the intervention group to the risk in the control group. A risk ratio of one indicates no difference between comparison groups. For undesirable outcomes, a risk ratio of less than one indicates that the intervention was effective in reducing the risk of that outcome.

Risk difference: Risk differences are the absolute difference in the event rate between two comparison groups. A risk difference of zero indicates no difference between comparison groups. For undesirable outcomes, a risk difference that is less than zero indicates that the intervention was effective in reducing the risk of that outcome.

Continuous data

Continuous data are outcomes that are summarised as means, arising through measurements or the use of assessment scales, and are summarised in systematic reviews as differences in means or standardised differences in mean (effect sizes).

Mean difference: Mean difference, as the name implies, is the difference between the means (i.e. the average values) of two groups.

Weighted mean difference: Weighted mean difference refers to the situation where studies have measured an outcome on the same scale, and the weight given to the mean difference in each study is usually equal to the inverse of the variance.

Standardised differences in mean: Standardised differences in mean refers to the situation where studies have measured an outcome using different scales or units of measurement (for example, inches and centimetres) and the mean difference may be divided by an estimate of the within group standard deviation to produce a standardised value without any units.

Effect measures

An effect measure is used to determine the extent to which outcomes are better or worse in the intervention group compared to the control group, and they are generated by comparing the outcomes of the two groups. When the effect measure has been established, it is possible to work out an average value across studies.

Meta-analysis may be carried out using either a 'fixed effect' or a 'random effects' model. Both are mathematical models for combining the results of studies. The fixed effect model assumes that the effect is truly constant in all of the populations studied. Thus, any variation within the study (referred to as 'within study' variation) is taken to influence the uncertainty of results and it produces narrower confidence intervals than the random effects model. The random effects model allows for variation in the effect amongst the populations studied. Thus, both within study variation and variation between studies (referred to as 'between study' variation) are included in the assessment of the uncertainty of results.

Data presentation

Generally speaking, results of synthesised data are presented in the form of a graph. There are several approaches used to achieve this including what is called a 'forest plot', which presents the individual study effects with their confidence intervals as horizontal lines and a box in the middle of that line representing the mean effect.

Qualitative data synthesis

According to Pearson (2004), the most complex problem in synthesising textual data is agreeing on and communicating techniques to compare the findings of the studies. Meta-synthesis relates to the combining of separate elements to form a coherent whole. This involves reasoning from the general to the particular using a process of interpretation. It is necessary for a reviewer of qualitative research evidence to establish certain criteria before carrying out data synthesis. These include:

- Rules for setting up categories
- How to assign findings to categories
- How to write narrative summaries for each category

All of these decisions need to be documented along with a rationale in the final systematic review report.

The analysis and synthesis of qualitative studies is based on processed data, just as with meta-analysis. There are, however, major differences between the approach used to synthesise the findings of randomised controlled trials and the approach used for qualitative studies.

Reality for the qualitative researcher, and reviewer, is viewed as multiple and constructed, and so undertaking meta-synthesis means that no two reviewers will produce exactly the same results. Although meta-synthesis provides only one interpretation, it aims to capture the essence of the phenomenon of interest.

When engaging in the synthesis of qualitative studies, differing research methods are not mixed in a single synthesis of all qualitative studies. The aim of meta-synthesis is to portray an accurate interpretation of a phenomenon and to compare and contrast the constructs of individual studies to reach consensus on a new construction of that phenomenon. Meta-synthesis involves the identification of findings, grouping findings into categories, and grouping those categories into synthesised findings.

Findings

Findings are conclusions reached by the researcher after examining the results of data analysis, often in the form of themes or metaphors. For instance, in our smoking example a finding might be:

While many descriptions could be interpreted as craving and nicotine withdrawal, patients perceived symptoms as signs of illness relapse.

And an illustration of that finding may be:

You have to keep a level up . . . like it's something your brain and body's doing automatically to let you know that your nicotine level is dropping . . . it's a physical thing of actually needing it.

Category

A category is a group of findings that reflects similar relationships between similar phenomena, variables or circumstances that may inform practice. For instance, in our smoking example a category might be:

Patients describe the use of cigarettes to deal with the physical symptoms of their illness.

Synthesis

Synthesised findings refer to the combining of separate elements to form a coherent whole, using logical deduction and reasoning from the general to the particular. For instance, in our smoking example a synthesis might be:

Smoking to self medicate illness.

These may be represented in the form of a diagram, such as that achieved in the JBI-QARI programme.

Learning activity

Data analysis or synthesis may or may not be possible for you at this point, depending on the types of studies you retrieved. Where possible, attempt to utilise the information and tools you now possess in order to perform either a meta-analysis or meta-synthesis. Where this is not possible, a narrative summary of the results in the studies identified may be required.

Practical tools for systematic reviews

There are several software programs available to assist in the systematic review process. These programs do not assist in making the methodological decisions that are required throughout the process, but are useful for tracking processes, critical appraisal, data extraction and analysis or synthesis.

Review Manager (RevMan)

The Cochrane Collaboration's computer program, commonly referred to as 'RevMan', was developed to assist in the preparation of that organisation's systematic reviews of effectiveness. The program allows a reviewer to enter protocols, perform meta-analysis of the data entered and present the results graphically using Meta View. RevMan is available for download from the Cochrane Collaboration at no cost to users.

System for the Unified Management of the Assessment and Review of Information (SUMARI)

The System for the Unified Management of the Assessment and Review of Information, or JBI-SUMARI, is a software suite designed to assist health and other researchers, scientists and practitioners to conduct systematic reviews of

Feasibility, Appropriateness, Meaningfulness and Effectiveness (FAME), and to conduct economic evaluations of activities and interventions. As with RevMan, SUMARI has a management component that manages the systematic review process, including protocol development. It also facilitates the critical appraisal, data extraction, data synthesis and report development processes. Each module interacts with the others and a reviewer may – at the point in the review when critical appraisal, data extraction and data synthesis/meta-analysis is reached – select a pathway to manage randomised control trials, non-randomised control trial quantitative data, qualitative data, textual data from opinion papers on reports, or economic data. SUMARI also consists of user groups and a bulletin board to enable users of the program to communicate with each other and the Institute.

Conclusion

Evidence, regardless of whether it is evidence of feasibility, appropriateness, meaningfulness or effectiveness, has the potential to influence health care practice in all disciplines. Research evidence is not always available on the interventions in which we might be interested; however, when it does exist it is important that it receives due consideration and that the quality of the research is determined prior to its utilisation in the clinical environment. Methods for appraising and analysing research evidence are consistently being reviewed and refined, but it is important to have a conceptual framework for these processes from which to start.

This chapter has examined the critical appraisal, data extraction and data analysis and synthesis of a wide variety of evidence for practice. It has also presented practical approaches to these important steps in the systematic review process. When reviewers have completed these steps, the next stage involves writing up the review report and developing guidelines to inform clinical practice.

In practice . . .

Having read about the processes of critical appraisal, data extraction and synthesis in considerable detail, think now about the benefits associated with health care professionals knowing how to perform these tasks and implement critically appraised evidence into their practice. What difference might this make to you in your own practice? If you have already experienced the clinical environment, think about a situation where you would use all forms of evidence in the clinical decision-making process. How do you think consumers of health care, such as Sarah, might benefit from having access to critically appraised evidence?

Further reading and resources

If you are interested in learning more about the material addressed in this chapter, we would suggest the following:

Alderson, P., Green, S., Higgins, J. P. T. (eds) (2003) Cochrane reviewers' handbook 4.2.2 [updated December 2003]. *The Cochrane Library 1*. Chichester, John Wiley & Sons Ltd.

Centre for Reviews and Dissemination (2001) Undertaking Systematic Reviews of Effectiveness. *CRD Report Number 4* (2nd edn). NHS Centre for Reviews and Dissemination, York.

Lemmer, B., Grellier, R. and Steven, J. (1999) Systematic review of non-random and qualitative research literature: exploring and uncovering an evidence base for health visiting and decision-making. *Qualitative Health Research* 9: 315–28.

Sandelowski, M., Docherty, S. and Emden, C. (1997) Qualitative meta-synthesis: issues and techniques. *Research in Nursing and Health* 20: 365–71.

Should you wish to undertake critical appraisal on single studies without performing any meta-analysis or synthesis of data, there are a couple of programs that may be of assistance:

Catmaker is focused on medical interventions but also includes diagnostic and prognostic risk studies and systematic reviews of intervention. Catnipper (a demonstration version of the Catmaker program) is available via the following link: www.cebm.net/cats.asp

RAPid is an online critical appraisal tool and training program designed to assist in the promotion of critical appraisal skills and research utilisation. It can organise, conduct and archive the findings of a single study or systematic review. RAPid is available via the following link: www.joannabriggs.edu.au/services/rapid.php

There are also several software packages available to assist in conducting systematic reviews. These include Review Manager (*RevMan*), developed by the Cochrane Collaboration, which manages the whole systematic review process. Review Manager is available free to download at: www.cc-ims.net/RevMan

The *SUMARI* software suite, developed by the Joanna Briggs Institute, is designed to assist reviewers in all components of the review process, from protocol development to critical appraisal, data extraction and synthesis of both quantitative and qualitative evidence. Further information on how to purchase the suite is available at: www.joannabriggs.edu.au

Chapter 7

Evidence Transfer: Writing up a Systematic Review Report and Developing Clinical Guidelines

'Example is not the main thing in influencing others, it is the only thing.' – Albert Schweitzer

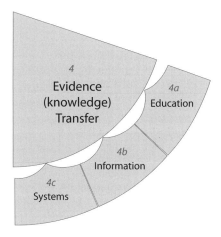

In Chapter 1 we explained the nature of evidence-based practice and the emergence and development of the evidence-based health care movement. In Chapter 2 we introduced the JBI Model of Evidence-Based Health Care and its components. In Chapter 3 we examined the nature of evidence and the various types of evidence that we consider to be useful for informing practice. In Chapter 4 we addressed the first of the substantive components of EBHC, which deals with the activity most fundamental to evidence-based practice, that is the generation of evidence. The basis of evidence-based practice is, of course, evidence. In Chapter 5 we moved on to the next component, that of the synthesis of evidence, and began to take you through the process of the systematic review. In so doing, we dealt only with the first half of the systematic review, locating the evidence. The second half of the systematic review process – the appraisal and evaluation of the evidence – we addressed in Chapter 6 where we took you through the processes and issues associated with the synthesis of different forms of evidence.

Now we progress a little further around the dial of the clock to the focus of this chapter, which is the next component of the JBI Model. This component, and thus this chapter, addresses the transfer of evidence. How do we disseminate the information gleaned during the systematic review? In the language of EBHC, this is referred to as evidence transfer and it entails a number of important elements that are addressed here. These elements include the writing up of the report of the systematic review. It may be possible to generate clinical guidelines from the outcomes of the systematic review and these too are addressed in this chapter.

This chapter focuses on evidence transfer and discusses:

- The systematic review report
- Clinical practice guidelines
- Rating the quality of the evidence
- Grading clinical practice guideline recommendations
- Developing clinical practice guidelines
- Appraising clinical practice guidelines

In practice . . .

A client named Robert, who has recently had cardiac surgery, has come into your care. He is well aware that he needs to quit smoking and has been planning on going cold turkey. The cravings, however, are already starting to get the better of him. You have now spent significant time and resources conducting a review of the evidence on smoking cessation and found that there are many interventions available to assist clients who wish to quit. None of these strategies has been established as the gold standard for success in quitting, but you believe that the information you have identified will be useful to individual practitioners and consumers like Robert in their decision-making processes.

As you read through this chapter, keep in mind Robert's situation. At various points you will be asked to think about how the content might relate to this case and whether it offers any solutions or strategies for assisting him.

Introduction

Most health professions are increasingly embracing the use of evidence-based guidelines to inform (rather than direct) practice, and this is a response to high-profile promotional initiatives of governments and provider agencies in individual countries. For example, in the US, considerable resources have been invested in high-quality, high-cost research and development programmes to develop clinical guidelines. The National Institutes of Health now have a well established strategy to review international literature and conduct meta-analyses to generate clinical guidelines based on best available evidence. Practical application of rigorously reviewed evidence is now promoted through the development and dissemination of practice guidelines in most developed health care systems. Clinical practice guidelines consist of statements to assist practitioner and patient decisions about appropriate health care for specific clinical circumstances, and are systematically developed on the basis of consensus within expert groups. An increasing number of well-constructed, practical and evidence-based guidelines are being developed, again largely within the US.

In the UK, recent policy initiatives have directed health care provider agencies to develop research and development (R & D) strategies, to establish R & D units and to promote practices based on best available knowledge. At the same time, the British government has established a number of centres for evidence-based practice, and health research centres such as the King's Fund support these.

There is also considerable international activity. For example, the Cochrane Collaboration has linked R & D sites across the world to review and analyse randomised clinical trials from an international perspective and to generate reports to inform practitioners, to influence practice and to be a resource in the development of consensus guidelines.

The purpose of the systematic review report

As we have seen in previous chapters, the core of evidence-based practice is the systematic review of the literature on a specific condition, intervention or issue. The systematic review is essentially an analysis of all the available literature and a judgement of the effectiveness or otherwise of a practice (see in particular Chapters 5 and 6).

The need for evidence to support clinical practice has never been greater. This need is the result of the vast array of available technologies and pharmaceutical and health care products. In addition, the body of knowledge upon which clinical practice is based is rapidly changing. Health professionals from all disciplines are required to make decisions as to which interventions, products and technologies should be implemented, and yet comparisons between products are often difficult because of limited information. Many of these health care products are also accompanied by sophisticated product promotion and claims of effectiveness, which also contribute to the difficulties when assessing their utility in the clinical environment.

Competition for health care resources has increased because of such things as increased consumer expectations, the ageing population and the ever-present threat of litigation when care provided does not meet expectations. The knowledge upon which health care is based is also changing rapidly and so some of what is taught to students will remain relevant for only a small portion of their professional careers. However, assisting health professionals to keep up to date with research and transferring this research evidence into practice has proven difficult.

While research, policy and practice have often seemed worlds apart, systematic review reports can provide a sound basis for clinical guidelines. Central to an evidence-based approach to clinical guideline development is the gathering and appraisal of the evidence in the form of a systematic review. Traditionally, as we have already discussed, this has been dominated by the systematic review of evidence of effectiveness. However, the types of evidence utilised to underpin clinical guidelines will vary (see Chapter 4) and it may be necessary to utilise different types of evidence for different aspects of a guideline for a specific intervention.

Writing the report

The components of the systematic review report will mirror to a certain extent the content of the original protocol. As with the protocol, there should be a **comprehensive background** that justifies conducting the review, a description of the **objectives of the review**, an account of the **criteria that were used for considering studies for the review**, the **search strategy used** and **methods utilised for critical appraisal, extraction and synthesis of data**.

The review of results should include a **description of the studies that includes the type and number of papers identified**. The number of papers that were included and excluded should be stated. There should also be a **summary of the overall quality of the literature identified**. The results section must be organised in a meaningful way, based on the objectives of the review and the criteria for considering studies. Particular consideration should be given to the types of interventions and outcomes. The reviewer should comment on the appropriateness of meta-view graphs in this section.

The **discussion** should include an **overview of the results** and it should **address issues arising from the conduct of the review including limitations and issues arising from the results of the review**. Conclusions should centre on **implications for practice** where possible. These should be detailed and must be based on the documented results, not author opinion. Where evidence is of a sufficient level, **appropriate recommendations** should also be made. Recommendations must be clear, concise and unambiguous. All implications for research must be derived from the results of the review.

Again, as in the initial protocol, the final review report should include references and appendices. The references should be appropriate in content and volume and include background references and studies from the initial search. The appendices should include:

- Critical appraisal form(s)
- Data extraction form(s)
- Table of included studies
- Table of excluded studies with justification for exclusion

These checklists should reflect the types of studies, settings, participants, interventions and outcomes for the review question posed. If systematic review reports are of a high enough standard, they may be utilised as evidence upon which to base clinical practice guidelines.

Learning activity

At this point you may wish to attempt writing up the work you have completed. Although not a full systematic review, this is an important part of the process worth practising. You might like to base the format upon that of the protocol and build your report from there.

What is a clinical guideline?

Clinical guidelines are sources of summarised information on specific practices related to patient care to guide health care professionals in their clinical decision-making. Guidelines are based on the best available evidence; they are designed to assist the practice of health care practitioners but do not replace their knowledge and skills.

Hutchinson and Baker (1999) argue strongly in favour of guidelines and suggest that good clinical guidelines can change the process of health care and improve outcomes. The authors also describe how, depending on the clinical questions being addressed, evidence can include systematic reviews; randomised controlled trials that examine effectiveness; economic analyses; representative epidemiological studies; and qualitative studies.

Significant work has been undertaken in recent years regarding guideline development and several agencies have been working towards the facilitation of evidence-based clinical guidelines for practice. These include organisations such as the National Institute for Health and Clinical Excellence (NICE), Scottish Intercollegiate Guidelines Network (SIGN), the Guidelines International Network (GIN), the Joanna Briggs Institute (JBI) and the Agency for Healthcare Quality and Research (AHQR).

NICE is an independent organisation responsible for providing national guidance on treatments and care for people using the NHS in England and Wales. Their guidance is intended for health care professionals, patients and their carers to help them make decisions about treatment and health care.

Similarly, the objective of SIGN is to improve the quality of health care for patients in Scotland by reducing variation in practice and outcome through the development and dissemination of national clinical guidelines containing recommendations for effective practice based on current evidence.

GIN seeks to improve the quality of health care by promoting systematic development of clinical practice guidelines and their application into practice through supporting international collaboration.

The Joanna Briggs Institute seeks to improve health outcomes and does so through the evaluation of evidence of effectiveness, appropriateness, meaningfulness and feasibility of health care practices and delivery methods.

In the United States, AHQR is a federal agency for research on health care quality, costs, outcomes and patient safety. AHQR produces a range of clinical guidelines and consumer information on a variety of interventions.

When preparing a guideline, the developers should formulate a series of questions to be answered. For example, a guideline may be written to clarify or resolve controversies, or to encourage more effective practice. According to Hutchinson and Baker (1999), there are four principal reasons for the increased interest in the development of guidelines:

- Shared clinical decision-making and increased teamwork
- The expanding evidence base of clinical practice
- The information technology revolution
- Inappropriate variation in clinical practice

Medicine-specific guidelines

Evidence-based medicine has, over the years, expanded rapidly from an idea into a movement, making a significant impact right across the broad field of health care to embrace nursing, health promotion, policy, management and a broad cross section of the allied health community. Evidence-based clinical guidelines have been an important vehicle for the transfer of evidence to practice.

Clinical guidelines for the medical profession have been controversial at times, particularly with regard to litigation. However, they are not, and were never intended to be, a substitute for professional discretion. Rather, they provide a summary of the best available evidence for clinicians to apply in specific contexts with individual clients.

Nursing-specific clinical guidelines

As stated previously, clinical guidelines are intended to provide health care staff with information, based on a systematic appraisal of the current best evidence, as to the optimum methods of addressing specific aspects of patient care. There are an increasing number of evidence-based, consensus guidelines for a wide range of health care practices. While clinical guidelines have been advocated for a considerable period of time, particularly in the medical profession, it is only in recent years that the wider health community has been able to access a more formalised process for the development and utilisation of evidence-based clinical practice guidelines.

Nursing in particular has made significant progress with the establishment of organisations dedicated to the generation of evidence-based clinical guidelines focused on nursing-specific interventions. Organisations such as the Joanna Briggs Institute in Australia and the Centre for Evidence-Based Nursing in the United Kingdom have been paramount in the evidence-based nursing movement. They have endeavoured to provide high-quality clinical guidelines that are reflective of the need to ground nursing in the beliefs, values and knowledge that underpin nursing practice as well as the use of the best available evidence.

Allied-health-specific guidelines

Conceptually, clinical practice guidelines are not new to the disciplines incorporated in the fields of allied health. However, the process of the systematic review of research evidence for the production of clinical guidelines is a relatively recent development. While these processes have been successfully initiated, allied health professionals face similar barriers to those medicine and nursing have experienced in the implementation of evidence-based practice. These include a perceived lack of time, lack of skills in evidence-based practice processes, organisational constraints, lack of relevant published evidence, and ambivalent attitudes towards evidence-based practice.

'Consensus' versus 'evidence'

While evidence-based practice has made substantial progress since its inception, there are often cases where 'best practice' is yet to be established, because of either a lack of 'generated' evidence or a lack of 'synthesised' evidence. In such situations, clinical expertise and professional opinion play a critically important role in health care decision-making.

Historically, where evidence has been used as a basis for guideline development, randomised controlled trials have predominated. However, given that many aspects of health care decision-making are not concerned with interventions and treatments susceptible of measurement by randomised controlled trials, the evidence available upon which to make decisions has been considered lacking. This has compelled guideline developers to seek information from other sources. Where evidence is not available, the subjective process of arriving at a recommendation for practice is usually based on professional opinion, experience, assumptions, beliefs and judgements.

It is anticipated that, with new developments in critical appraisal of other forms of evidence for inclusion in systematic reviews of research, the inclusion of consensus may diminish somewhat. In the meantime guidelines will no doubt involve a combination of evidence and consensus, but it should be ensured that the processes behind the development of such guidelines are explicit and transparent so that clinicians can clearly distinguish between those recommendations based on consensus and those based on the best available evidence (and the quality of that evidence should also be explicit).

Upon completion, systematic reviews of the best available evidence can be utilised to develop clinical guidelines on specific practices related to patient care to guide health care professionals in their clinical practice, making evidence *meaningful* in the clinical environment.

Decision toolkit

Decision	Tools	Evaluation
How to make the evidence useful for health professionals and consumers.	A solid approach to systematically reviewing the evidence and a multidisciplinary approach to guideline development.	Were you able to provide Robert with evidence-based health information on smoking cessation?

Strategies for guideline development

The continued development and innovation in the evidence-based movement means that access to valid and reliable research upon which to base clinical guidelines is better than ever. Guideline developers are now not only able to base guidelines on a comprehensive synthesis of the international evidence, but are now moving toward a more explicit process for development of guidelines and recommendations.

A definitive attribute of clinical guidelines for health care professionals is their foundation on research evidence. Historically, guidelines have often been consensus based, but as we have already established, practice should be based on the best available evidence. As mentioned in previous chapters, this evidence may be generated through a variety of research methods as well as through expert opinion. The identification, appraisal and synthesis of relevant research upon which to base guidelines and recommendations for practice has been discussed in previous chapters. However, these processes represent what is largely a technical or academic process. The formulation of guidelines is far more involved and it is often considered to be somewhat controversial as it revolves, to a certain extent, around the interpretation of evidence in order to make decisions regarding clinical practice and policy.

It is for this reason that both the recommendation, and the evidence upon which it is based, is graded in terms of quality and strength. Evidence should be translated into clinically useful recommendations, and those recommendations should be based on the highest level of evidence. However, evidence alone is insufficient when making recommendations for practice. Developers are required to use their judgement, experience and good sense for translating evidence into recommendations that are going to be clinically useful. In order to achieve this, the development group should be multidisciplinary and where possible consumers should also be involved in this process. The preferences of both the health practitioner and the consumer are vital to the successful development and implementation of any clinical guideline.

Rarely is a health care intervention isolated to one discipline, and stakeholders can assist in identifying relevant outcomes, values and target audiences, and indeed, they can assist in identifying potential obstacles to implementation. Guidelines should be flexible and adaptable, and therefore it is important to determine whether the evidence is relevant to different target populations and whether it is appropriate to the geographical and clinical setting.

The process of implementing a new clinical guideline may present organisational challenges with regard to financial burden. In times of economic stringency in health care, health professionals wishing to implement clinical change must present a strong case, and so guidelines should be developed with resource constraints in mind. It is therefore important to take into account whether there are appropriate economic studies available, and where possible, an economic appraisal should be conducted. Economic evidence may impact on the feasibility of the intervention, making it a consideration of significant consequence.

Guidelines should also take into account their target audience. There is no single format for the presentation of guidelines. A broad range of presentation styles is available and guidelines can be produced in a variety of forms and formats to meet the specific needs of multiple target groups. These might include a compilation of short summaries for use in professional or general publications, brochures, posters, the internet, audio or videotapes, or on disk or CD-ROM. Any combination of approaches may be utilised, provided that the final product is explicit, logical, clear and succinct and that dissemination strategies are tailored to the specific target group. Dissemination alone, however, will not change the behaviour of health professionals or consumers, and this will be addressed in the following chapter.

Guidelines should be revised regularly, and therefore both the evidence and the recommendations arising from them should be dated and an intended date for revision given. Evaluation and revision of guidelines should consider the following (NHMRC, 1999):

- How well were the guidelines disseminated?
- Is the general trend in clinical practice moving towards the guideline recommendations?
- Have the guidelines contributed to any specific changes in clinical practice?
- How have the guidelines affected consumers' knowledge and understanding?
- Have health outcomes changed?

The guideline process should also be subjected to an economic evaluation in order to assess all of the costs incurred in providing the guideline and assessing its impact. The guidelines' relevance, accessibility, usability and content clarity should also be assessed.

Learning activity

Although at this stage you have not completed a full systematic review of the evidence on your field of interest, think about the process you have worked through thus far and how this process, and the resulting information, might be utilised in the clinical environment. Then think about how you might go about informing practice with this information. Who are the key stakeholders and how will they benefit from the information you have generated? For instance, how might Robert benefit from equivalent information pertinent to his situation?

The quality of the evidence

Conceptually, levels of evidence and grades of recommendation have evolved in recent years, most distinctively in terms of the differentiation between the two. The utility of information generated from conducting systematic reviews relies quite substantially on the existence of a system for grading the evidence. This process is an important element when making recommendations for practice in order to enable health professionals to distinguish recommendations based on consensus from those based on good-quality studies with consistent findings (Hutchinson and Baker, 1999).

While there are a number of generally accepted ranking scales used to categorise evidence in terms of quality, there is yet to be an agreed international standard.

Hutchinson and Baker (1999) suggest that grading of evidence statements in guidelines should be readily understandable as their function is to alert the casual reader or busy clinician to the strength or weakness of specific statements.

Table 7.1 Three-point level of evidence scale.

Level 1: Good	Evidence includes consistent results from well-designed, well-conducted studies in representative populations that directly assess effects on health outcomes.
Level 2: Fair	Evidence is sufficient to determine effects on health outcomes, but the number, quality, or consistency of the individual studies, generalisability to routine practice, or indirect nature of the evidence on health outcomes limits the strength of the evidence.
Level 3: Poor	Evidence is insufficient to assess the effects on health outcomes because of limited number or power of studies, important flaws in their design or conduct, gaps in the chain of evidence, or lack of information on important health outcomes.

Many organisations utilise a three-point scale, as in Table 7.1. However, such scales are not always reflective of the breadth of research evidence. In order to accommodate such differences in evidence, several more complex scales have been developed, including one by the Centre for Evidence-Based Medicine in Oxford, UK (Table 7.2).

This hierarchy takes a broad view of evidence. There is general agreement internationally that the randomised controlled trial represents the 'gold standard' in evidence of effectiveness but there are a large number of evidence hierarchies in use by the numerous evidence review groups. There is considerable variation in approaches to evidence tables in terms of levels and when they should be used.

The international debate about evidence tables is vigorous and although there is no consensus the trend is toward revisiting the use of grades of recommendation. As an international collaboration, with an interest in expanding the definition of evidence to include evidence of feasibility, appropriateness, meaningfulness and economic impact, the Joanna Briggs Institute adopted the evidence hierarchy in Table 7.3 in 2004. Systematic reviewers with expertise in research methods use levels of evidence to determine the quality of evidence. Grades of recommendation are often used in abstracted evidence, evidence summaries or clinical guidelines.

Grades of recommendation

There is little point in accumulating evidence to answer a question if we cannot then use that answer to develop recommendations to benefit patients. Critically, evidence-based practice involves the integration of best available evidence with clinical expertise to improve health outcomes. When it comes to deciding whether or not to incorporate into practice a particular activity or intervention, some or all of the following considerations will be relevant:

- Is it available?
- Is it affordable?

Table 7.2 Oxford Centre for Evidence-Based Medicine Levels of Evidence.

Level	Therapy/prevention, aetiology/harm	Prognosis	Diagnosis	Differential diagnosis/symptom prevalence study	Economic and decision analyses
1a	SR (with homogeneity) of RCTs	SR (with homogeneity) of inception cohort studies; CDR† validated in different populations	SR (with homogeneity) of Level 1 diagnostic studies; CDR with 1b studies from different clinical centres	SR (with homogeneity) of prospective cohort studies	SR (with homogeneity) of Level 1 economic studies
1b	Individual RCT (with narrow confidence interval)	Individual inception cohort study with >80% follow-up; CDR† validated in a single population	Validating cohort study with good reference standards; or CDR tested within one clinical centre	Prospective cohort study with good follow-up	Analysis based on clinically sensible costs or alternatives; systematic review(s) of the evidence; and including multi-way sensitivity analyses
1c	All or none	All or none case-series	Absolute SpPins and SnNouts	All or none case-series	Absolute better-value or worse-value analyses
2a	SR (with homogeneity) of cohort studies	SR (with homogeneity) of either retrospective cohort studies or untreated control groups in RCTs	SR (with homogeneity) of Level >2 diagnostic studies	SR (with homogeneity) of 2b and better studies	SR (with homogeneity) of Level >2 economic studies
2b	Individual cohort study (including low quality RCT; e.g., <80% follow-up)	Retrospective cohort study or follow-up of untreated control patients in an RCT; Derivation of CDR or validated on split-sample only	Exploratory cohort study with good reference standards; CDR after derivation, or validated only on split-sample or databases	Retrospective cohort study, or poor follow-up	Analysis based on clinically sensible costs or alternatives; limited review(s) of the evidence, or single studies; and including multi-way sensitivity analyses
2c	'Outcomes' research; Ecological studies	'Outcomes' research		Ecological studies	Audit or outcomes research
3a	SR (with homogeneity) of case-control studies		SR (with homogeneity) of 3b and better studies	SR (with homogeneity) of 3b and better studies	SR (with homogeneity) of 3b and better studies
3b	Individual case-control study		Non-consecutive study; or without consistently applied reference standards	Non-consecutive cohort study, or very limited population	Analysis based on limited alternatives or costs, poor quality estimates of data, but including sensitivity analyses incorporating clinically sensible variations.
4	Case-series (and poor quality cohort and case-control studies)	Case-series (and poor quality prognostic cohort studies)	Case-control study, poor or non-independent reference standard	Case-series or superseded reference standards	Analysis with no sensitivity analysis
5	Expert opinion without explicit critical appraisal, or based on physiology, bench research or 'first principles'	Expert opinion without explicit critical appraisal, or based on physiology, bench research or 'first principles'	Expert opinion without explicit critical appraisal, or based on physiology, bench research or 'first principles'	Expert opinion without explicit critical appraisal, or based on physiology, bench research or 'first principles'	Expert opinion without explicit critical appraisal, or based on economic theory or 'first principles'

Produced by Bob Phillips, Chris Ball, Dave Sackett, Doug Badenoch, Sharon Straus, Brian Haynes, Martin Dawes since November 1998
http://www.cebm.net/levels_of_evidence.asp#levels. SR = systematic review; CDR = clinical decision rule; RCT = randomised controlled trial.

Table 7.3 The Joanna Briggs Institute Levels of Evidence.

Level of Evidence	Feasibility F(1–4)	Appropriateness A(1–4)	Meaningfulness M(1–4)	Effectiveness E(1–4)	Economic Evidence EE(1–4)
1	SR of research with unequivocal synthesised findings	SR of research with unequivocal synthesised findings	SR of research with unequivocal synthesised findings	SR (with homogeneity) of experimental studies (e.g. RCT with concealed allocation) or one or more large experimental studies with narrow confidence intervals	SR (with homogeneity) of evaluations of important alternative interventions comparing all clinically relevant outcomes against appropriate cost measurement, and including a clinically sensible sensitivity analysis
2	SR of research with credible synthesised findings	SR of research with credible synthesised findings	SR of research with credible synthesised findings	Quasi-experimental studies (e.g. without randomisation)	Evaluation of important alternative interventions comparing all clinically relevant outcomes against appropriate cost measurement, and including a clinically sensible sensitivity analysis
3	SR of text/opinion with credible synthesised findings	SR of text/opinion with credible synthesised findings	SR of text/opinion with credible synthesised findings	3a. Cohort studies (with control group) 3b. Case-controlled 3c Observational studies without control groups	Evaluation of important alternative interventions comparing a limited number of outcomes against appropriate cost measurement, without a clinically sensible sensitivity analysis
4	Expert opinion without explicit critical appraisal	Expert opinion without explicit critical appraisal	Expert opinion without explicit critical appraisal	Expert opinion without explicit critical appraisal, or based on physiology, bench research or consensus	Expert opinion without explicit critical appraisal, or based on economic theory

- Is it applicable in the setting?
- Would the patient/client be a willing participant in the implementation of the intervention?
- Were the patients in the study or studies that provided the evidence sufficiently similar to your own to justify the implementation of this particular intervention?
- What will be the potential benefits for the patient?
- What will be the potential harms for the patient?
- Does this intervention allow for the individual patient's values and preferences?

As well as needing to define levels of evidence for practice, it is also necessary to utilise grades of recommendations for practice. Again, there are numerous examples of how recommendations can be graded. Table 7.4 shows a fairly typical approach to this exercise, drawing from evidence that has previously been ranked in terms of level.

Pearson (2004) states that current approaches to evaluating evidence utilise a hierarchy of evidence designed to assess the validity of recommendations for clinical guidelines. These approaches focus on effectiveness of treatment and rank only quantitative evidence according to the rigour of the research, that is the extent to which it is designed to limit bias. More recently, with attempts being made to be more inclusive of other forms of evidence, new scales are being developed to reflect this progress. Among such efforts to categorise the validity of qualitative evidence is the FAME scale, described by Pearson (2002) (Table 7.5) as a hierarchy of *applicability* of evidence used to grade recommendations by the Joanna Briggs Institute.

Table 7.4 Grades of recommendation: these recommendation grades reflect the strength of evidence and magnitude of net benefit (benefits minus harms).

A	Strongly recommend that clinicians adopt this. Good evidence found to suggest that this improves important health outcomes and the benefits substantially outweigh the harms.
B	Recommend that clinicians adopt this. At least fair evidence found to suggest that it improves important health outcomes and that the benefits outweigh the harms.
C	No recommendation for or against adoption. At least fair evidence that it can improve health outcomes but the balance of benefits and harms is too close to justify a general recommendation.
D	Recommend against routinely adopting this. At least fair evidence found that suggests that it is ineffective or that harms outweigh benefits.
I	The evidence is insufficient to recommend for or against routinely adopting this. Evidence that it is effective is lacking, of poor quality, or conflicting and the balance of benefits and harms cannot be determined.

Adapted from US Preventive Services Task Force (USPSTF): www.ahcpr.gov/clinic/uspst-fix.htm (accessed 17 March 2004).

Table 7.5 Levels of applicability of evidence.

Grade of recommendation	Feasibility	Appropriateness	Meaningfulness	Effectiveness
A	Immediately practicable	Ethically acceptable and justifiable	Provides a strong rationale for practice change	Effectiveness established to a degree that merits application
B	Practicable with limited training and/or modest additional resources	Ethical acceptance is unclear	Provides a moderate rationale for practice change	Effectiveness established to a degree that suggests application
C	Practicable with significant additional training and/or resources	Conflicts to some extent with ethical principles	Provides limited rationale for practice change	Effectiveness established to a degree that warrants consideration of applying the findings
D	Practicable with extensive additional training and/or resources	Conflicts considerably with ethical principles	Provides minimal rationale for advocating change	Effectiveness established to a limited degree
E	Impracticable	Ethically unacceptable	There is no rationale to support practice change	Effectiveness not established

---

Learning activity

Think about the information you have identified thus far and how you might grade the quality of that evidence. Having given this some thought, how do you now think that evidence might impact on practice?

Consumer involvement in guideline development

Consumer involvement in clinical guideline development has long been advocated, although there is little documented research regarding how and when to involve consumers and what to expect from them within the process of guideline development (Eccles et al., 2000). Consumer involvement in clinical guideline development is important as consumers have the potential to bring a rich source of knowledge, understanding and experience to this process that is quite different from that of the health professional.

There are many strategies available for consumer involvement, some of which have proven more successful than others. Some groups have utilised methods that incorporate an individual consumer on a guideline development panel; others have taken a more comprehensive approach that involves conducting a series of workshops with relevant consumer groups to explore the potential of increasing patients' understanding of the meaning of scientific evidence, their ideas of cost-effectiveness and their views on patient information.

Bastian (1996) argues that if consumer involvement is to successfully raise the standard of health care guidelines, then the standard of consumer participation itself needs to be raised. She recommends that consumer involvement should be both within guideline development groups and in other structures outside of guideline development groups that feed into them.

Guideline appraisal

Clinical guidelines have been recognised as one of the most promising and effective advances for defining and improving the quality of care. However, it is essential that the validity, reliability, reproducibility and transparency of guidelines be well established. The percentage of available guidelines that currently meet appraisal criteria is questionable, and thus there is a necessity for the establishment of documents, such as technical reports, that provide information regarding the process used for development of the guideline.

There are several checklists and tools available for the critical appraisal of clinical practice guidelines. One such tool is the 'Appraisal of Guidelines Research and Evaluation' (AGREE). It originates from an international collaboration of researchers and policy makers who work together to improve the quality and effectiveness of clinical practice guidelines by establishing a shared framework for their development, reporting and assessment.

The AGREE instrument is a generic guideline appraisal checklist that focuses on the following.

Scope and purpose:

- The overall objective(s) of the guideline should be specifically described.
- The clinical question(s) covered by the guideline should be specifically described.
- The patients to whom the guideline is meant to apply should be specifically described.

Stakeholder involvement:

- The guideline development group should include individuals from all the relevant professional groups.
- The patient's views and preferences should be sought.

Rigour of development:

- Systematic methods should be used to search for evidence.
- The criteria for selective evidence should be clearly described.
- The methods for formulating the recommendations should be clearly described.

- The health benefits, side effects and risks should be considered in formulating the recommendations.
- There should be an explicit link between the recommendations and the supporting evidence.
- The guideline should be externally reviewed by experts prior to publication.
- A procedure for updating the guideline should be provided.

Clarity and presentation:

- The recommendations should be specific and unambiguous.
- The different options for diagnosis and/or treatment of the condition should be clearly presented.
- Key recommendations should be easily identifiable.

Applicability:

- The target users of the guideline should be clearly defined.
- The potential organisational barriers in applying the recommendations should be discussed.
- The potential cost implications of applying the recommendations should be considered.
- The guideline should be supported with tools for application.
- The guideline should present key review criteria for monitoring and audit purposes.
- The guideline should be piloted among end users.

Editorial independence:

- The guideline should be editorially independent from the funding body.
- Conflicts of interest of guideline developers should be recorded.

Learning activity

Find an existing guideline specific to your area of practice. Now using the AGREE tool, go through the process of appraising that guideline. Does it meet all of the criteria on this list to your satisfaction? You may wish to try this on several guidelines to determine the extent of variability in quality. Try to locate a guideline that may assist with Robert's cessation of smoking. If you are successful in locating such a guideline, subject it, too, to the AGREE appraisal.

The role of guidelines in practice

The goal of clinical guidelines is to improve the quality of health care received by patients and, in turn, to improve health outcomes. However, clinical guidelines are used only intermittently in health care practice and the enormous amount of time and energy spent on their development is of little use if they have no impact on practice.

The role of guidelines in clinical practice is threefold and encompasses the implementation of research evidence into practice, policy development and revision, and direct care provision for patients.

The first of these is concerned essentially with encouraging the utilisation of research evidence in the clinical environment. It has been clear for some time now that one of the greatest barriers to improving the effectiveness of health care is the difficulty faced by health professionals in getting research into practice. Indeed, this is a central preoccupation of Chapter 8. One of the key functions of clinical practice guidelines is as a practical tool for the assimilation of new research evidence into practice. Guidelines may also contribute to the process of optimising health care resources and influencing health care policy.

Finally, guidelines may be utilised to enhance decision-making processes not only for health professionals but also for consumers of health care. Several guideline development organisations have initiated processes to enhance communication with consumers by translating clinical practice guidelines into plain English for the benefit of patients, carers and families involved in the decision-making process.

Practical tools for guideline development

The role and nature of guidelines has been explained in this chapter, as has the process through which they are developed. It will be obvious from this discussion that there are many resources accessible to health care professionals who wish to embark upon the process of developing guidelines. For example, the material relating to methodology of guideline development known as SIGN 50 is readily available on the SIGN website and is an excellent place to start.

The Guidelines International Network (GIN) also has an excellent array of resources for those who wish to develop guidelines. According to their website (April 2005), they offer their members the following:

- Access to the International Guideline Library. This gives members of GIN the capacity to search and review the programmes for guidelines, systematic review, evidence reports and guideline clearing reports of all member organisations.
- **Development tools and resources** that provide information about the latest techniques and instruments for developing evidence-based guidelines.
- **Training materials** for producing and using clinical practice guidelines.
- **Patient/consumer resources** from members of GIN.
- **Guidelines from those who are not members** of GIN.
- Access to the **health topics collection** with guidelines for specific health topics.

It is also worthwhile bearing in mind that the AHQR hosts the National Guidelines Clearing House and provides a set of 'Quality Tools', which are accessible via its website; and the Joanna Briggs Institute website has online libraries of systematic reviews, technical reports, best practice information sheets, evidence summaries and evidence-based guides for practice.

Conclusion

Many health professionals in a variety of clinical settings are faced with the challenges posed by incorporating evidence-based practice into health care. As the nature of clinical practice changes and clinical guidelines evolve, health professionals will be required to adapt also. However, regardless of circumstance, guidelines should remain pertinent and relevant to their local context.

The NHMRC (2000) asserts that the key issue is that a decision has to be made about what is feasible and appropriate in a given situation and the extent to which reasonable standards have been met by the available body of evidence.

This chapter has examined the importance of reporting the results of the systematic review process and developing guidelines for practice. The challenge remains, however, regarding the successful implementation and utilisation of clinical guidelines in the clinical practice environment. The issues surrounding this will be addressed in the following chapter along with some practical tools and strategies for implementation.

In practice . . .

Your involvement in the guideline development process may be basic (appraisal of guidelines for relevance to your clinical context) or advanced (participation in guideline development groups and implementation teams). While many health professionals may not be personally involved in guideline development, they will often be faced with guidelines that they are supposed to utilise in their practice, so it is important for them to be able to note the difference between consensus and evidence as a basis for guidelines; note the steps in guideline development; and consider the role of guidelines in their own practice.

Select three guidelines that are related to your area of practice and think about whether they are useful to practitioners, whether they reflect practice and whether you believe the recommendations being made.

Having worked your way through this chapter and after considering the three guidelines of relevance to your area, do you believe that clinical guidelines would have anything to offer in assisting Robert to quit smoking?

Further reading and resources

If you would like to read more about the development and implementation of clinical practice guidelines, the following titles may be of interest:

Conroy, M. and Shannon, W. (1995) Clinical guidelines: their implementation in general practice. British Journal of General Practice **45**: 371–5.
Dunn, E., Norton, P., et al. (1994) Disseminating research/changing practice. In: *Research Methods for Primary Care* Vol 6. Thousand Oaks, CA, Sage Publications.

NHMRC (1999) *A Guide to the Development, Implementation and Evaluation of Clinical Practice Guidelines*. Canberra, National Health and Medical Research Council.

If you would like to find out more about guideline development and the organisations that are involved in the process of guideline development, the following websites may be of interest:

Agency for Healthcare Research and Quality: www.ahcpr.gov/clinic/uspstfix.htm
Guidelines International Network: www.nice.org.uk/page.aspx?o=206320
Joanna Briggs Institute: www.joannabriggs.edu.au
National Institute for Health and Clinical Excellence: www.nice.org.uk/
Scottish Intercollegiate Guidelines Network: www.sign.ac.uk/

Chapter 8

Evidence Utilisation: Implementing Evidence-Based Guidelines

'Change has a considerable psychological impact on the human mind. To the fearful it is threatening because it means that things may get worse. To the hopeful it is encouraging because things may get better. To the confident it is inspiring because the challenge exists to make things better.' – *Whitney King Jnr*

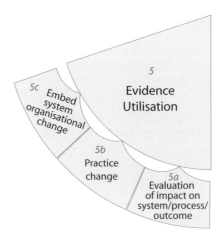

In Chapter 1 we explained the nature of evidence-based practice and the emergence and development of the evidence-based health care movement. In Chapter 2 we introduced the JBI Model of Evidence-Based Health Care and its components. In Chapter 3 we examined the nature of evidence and the various types of evidence that we consider to be useful for informing practice. In Chapter 4 we addressed the first of the substantive components of EBHC, which deals with the activity most fundamental to evidence-based practice, that is the generation of evidence. In Chapter 5 we moved on to the next component, that of the synthesis of evidence and began to take you through the process of the systematic review. We concluded our treatment of the systematic review in Chapter 6 where we took you through the processes and issues associated with the synthesis of different forms of evidence. In Chapter 7 we considered the transfer of evidence, dwelling primarily on the reporting of the systematic review and the development of clinical guidelines.

In Chapter 8 we consider how to implement these evidence-based clinical guidelines into practice. The emphasis here is on change and its management, along with an extensive consideration of the barriers to change, since it is these that are primarily responsible for the limited uptake of evidence into practice.

This chapter focuses on evidence utilisation and discusses:

- Leading and managing change
- Change theories
- Change strategies
- Overcoming barriers to change

In practice . . .

You have established what is best practice and developed clinical guidelines for the cessation of smoking, but other members of staff have shown significant resistance to implementation. They see nothing wrong with the interventions that have been promoted in the past and they simply do not have the time to spend on educating clients about smoking cessation. They have far more important clinical work that requires their attention. You decide to raise the issue with your manager to see if there might be any strategies that could be used to implement the smoking cessation guideline. Management has accepted the revised protocol for the assessment, treatment, consultation and documentation of clients who are having difficulty in quitting smoking. However, your continued efforts to encourage other staff members to follow it have been unsuccessful.

As you read through this chapter, keep in mind this scenario. At various points you will be asked to think about how the content of the chapter might relate to this case and whether it offers any solutions or strategies for achieving the goal of changing practice for smoking cessation in this facility.

Introduction

The systematic review of evidence and development of clinical guidelines pose significant challenges for health professionals in the practical setting. Evidence-based practice necessitates guideline development, education and review in order to achieve improved clinical outcomes. However, initiatives that endeavour to disseminate and implement clinical practice guidelines have often faced significant barriers and opposition, such as restricted access to information, environmental factors, professional inertia and perceived degrees of usefulness or uselessness! (See Hutchinson and Baker, 1999.)

We would argue that the ultimate success of the evidence-based movement is dependent upon the degree to which it has an impact on health service outcomes. Nursing provides good examples of why this is so. Theories for developing practice in the past, such as the nursing process and models of nursing, have failed this litmus test and lost both momentum and credibility. Despite considerable efforts to persuade clinicians and adapt theories to practice, clinicians were reluctant to change. The study of change is an integral element in the implementation phase of evidence-based practice.

The transfer of evidence into practice is often at best slow, and the process can be intractably difficult for a range of complex reasons. Thus, a coordinated strategy requiring appropriate skill, determination, time, money and planning is prudent for the success of any programme of implementation. In Australia, the National Health & Medical Research Council (NHMRC, 2000) suggest that there are four elements that are desirable in order for the successful transfer of research evidence to occur. These include good information based on research that is capable of standing up to rigorous critical appraisal and that will assist in solving practical problems; effective mechanisms and strategies for dissemination that enable health professionals and consumers to access information; physical and intellectual environments in which research is valued and uptake of research-based knowledge is supported and encouraged; and interventions that demonstrably promote the uptake of knowledge and lead to behaviour change.

In this chapter we will review some of the theory behind the change process. We will identify the key stakeholders involved and their contribution to the change process, along with some practical tools and strategies for effective practice change. However, we will begin with a consideration of the barriers to change because acknowledging and understanding these barriers is critical to the successful implementation of change.

> **In practice . . .**
>
> If you have ever attempted to achieve change in practice at an organisational level or just among your colleagues, take a few minutes to reflect on that experience. Was it successful? If so, consider what factors may have contributed to that success. Similarly, if it was unsuccessful, what factors contributed to failure?

Barriers to change

There is sometimes the assumption that in order to improve care, clinicians primarily need more concise information and user-friendly formats and systems to help them apply research findings and evidence-based guidelines. However, there is a need to address not only the information requirements of health professionals and organisations but also the social and organisational factors that interfere with the application of research findings.

Regardless of profession or discipline, any plan for change requires the ability to overcome barriers to its successful implementation. These barriers may occur at different levels, regardless of whether it is organisational, staff or consumer driven, and the barriers will vary considerably for the stakeholders involved. A variety of strategies are available to overcome such barriers, and that is why it is imperative that they are identified prior to initiating any approach to facilitating change. This may be achieved through the utilisation of surveys, interviews or focus groups involving all key stakeholders. The aim is to elicit their perspectives on the proposed change and to provide the stakeholders with an opportunity to feel ownership for that change.

It is important to identify potential barriers to change in the local context, and there may be characteristics of the proposed change that have the potential to influence its adoption. For example, it may be necessary to pilot the change in order to assess whether or not it is compatible with current beliefs and practices of the context, as well as whether health professionals in the target group are open to the possibility of change.

Other potential external barriers to implementation of evidence-based practice might include inadequate access to information, insufficient time and money to acquire new skills, low levels of baseline skills in critical appraisal, problems with the medical and nursing hierarchy, perceived threats to medical autonomy, or lack of evidence.

If it is possible, identify those issues or problems that may make it difficult to develop evidence-based practice, and then try to identify an equal number of points that assist the process. When a number of barriers and enablers have been identified, a useful strategy might be to discuss them with the clinical team to see if there are ways of using the enabling factors and if there are any ways around the blocking factors. In the event that those blocking factors prove to be insurmountable, the most constructive approach may be to abandon that particular project and move on to another.

For example, a clinical audit might be conducted where the staff identify seven areas of concern in the prevention of falls by residents. They may be successful in changing five of those areas of concern, but it may be that management is unable to afford the costs associated with the last two. The staff will have improved the things that lay within their power and might comfortably move on to audit a new topic.

Some of the most common barriers to change include the following.

Staff information and skill deficit: A common barrier to evidence-based practice that is listed by health professionals is information and skill deficit. Lack of knowledge regarding the indications and/or contraindications, current recommendations and guidelines, or results of clinical research have the potential to cause health professionals to feel that they do not have sufficient technical training, skill or expertise to implement the change.

Psychosocial barriers: Psychosocial barriers are also common in situations where change is imminent. The feelings, attitudes, beliefs, values and previous experiences of staff that affect clinical practice will play a considerable role during the change period.

Organisational barriers: Organisational, structural and systemic limitations may also prove to be significant barriers to change. These may include anything from outdated standing orders or accountability gaps through to the mode of resource allocation.

Resource barriers: Appropriate and effective patient care may not be achieved if the required tools, equipment, staff and other resources required to successfully achieve are not available.

Patient knowledge/skill barriers: Patients, their families or their carers may lack knowledge or information that is necessary for successful treatment, and this may present a barrier to the proposed change.

Patient psychosocial barriers and preferences: Patients and/or their families may hold feelings, beliefs, values and experiences that interfere with successful treatment, and these may present a barrier to the proposed change.

In practice . . .

Before moving on to consider how practice can be changed, consider the impact of the barriers to change that you have just read through. These barriers imply that change is well nigh impossible to achieve. Why is it, then, that just sometimes change – even major change – is achieved with a minimum of fuss and bother?

Changing practice

Leading and managing change

Changing health care practice is essentially bringing about an alteration in behaviour or substituting one way of behaviour for another. Some changes occur because of things around us, but most changes cannot effectively occur without being planned. Planned change is inevitably easier to manage than change that is imposed, haphazard or misunderstood. Health care professionals are agents of change. They frequently endeavour to bring about changes in the behaviour of clients, such as changing dependence into independence, fear into feelings of security and so forth.

Although now something of a cliché, it is true that change is a part of our everyday lives. Is it, then, a quirk of human nature that causes us to resist that which is known to be inevitable? In order to understand and work around resistance to change, it is helpful for leaders to consider resistance as a fundamental component of the change process. An understanding of why people resist, and ways in which resistance is manifested, can go some way towards helping health care professionals to lead and to smooth the path of change. It is therefore an important prerequisite to planning.

Resistance is commonly viewed in two ways:

- Resistance effectively hampers and blocks change.
- Resistance maintains order and stability.

Resistance can thus be considered to be both good and bad: bad in terms of preventing or blocking something that may be advantageous or even essential; good in terms of tempering and balancing, thus constituting a brake on unplanned change.

One of the most effective ways of minimising resistance is to actively involve people at all stages of the process. Giving people the opportunity to contribute and become part of the change personally engages them and offers them the chance to help rather than hinder. It can create a feeling of worth and recognition. As in all negotiations, the achievement of those things that we consider essential will often involve trading off those things that we consider less important.

Response to change is also concerned with emotional reactions. The emotional cycle of the change process, described by Kelley and Connor (1979), relates to the feelings experienced by people participating in change (Figure 8.1). As they point out, 'emotions of the participants fluctuate from highs to lows, and it would appear that these "highs" and "lows" can be identified with particular stages in the change process'. Although now somewhat dated, this work still rings true to the experience of the majority of change agents. They go on to describe this cycle in the following way:

'Things usually start off with a "high", before the participants become fully aware of what they are really letting themselves in for. This stage is referred to as uninformed optimism. The stage of informed pessimism begins when people begin to recognise the full implications, and perhaps come up against problems. This is the point at which some participants may even wish to withdraw so plans need to be laid to help them through. However, with acknowledgement, support and perhaps some re-structuring hope will begin to be generated. This is the stage of hopeful realism. Hope, and some evidence of a return for the efforts that have been made, instil confidence in the venture. This is known as the stage of informed optimism and sees the participants through to rewarding completion, which brings the glow of satisfaction.'

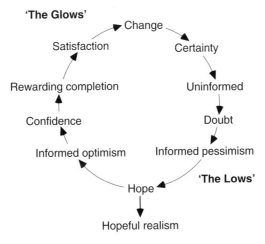

Fig. 8.1 The emotional response to change (adapted from Kelley and Connor, 1979).

Learning activity

It is well established that change is not an easy process. Whether we are changing where we live, changing our diet or exercise routine, or changing our approach to aspects of our work, 'change' usually equates to 'challenge'. Think about an aspect of your life (whether work or personally oriented) to which you were required to make a significant change. How did you approach the change? How did it make you feel? What strategies did you employ to overcome the challenge of that change? And how might you approach change in the future, having learned from your experience?

Evidence-based health care and practice change

Throughout this text it has been suggested that contemporary practice is rarely based on the best available evidence; thus, implementing an evidence-based approach represents a major change in health care. This is recognised by many health professionals internationally.

Medicine

The hostility of medicine toward change, it has been suggested, has been a product of concerns regarding the potential threat to professional autonomy of individual practitioners, rationing of health care and the idea that evidence-based medicine presents a distorted or partial view of science and rejects much that is central to the scientific method. Although evidence-based medicine has made an enormous impact on health care education and policy, its translation into practice has not been universally accepted and the integration of the principles of evidence-based practice has been as inconsistent as for other health disciplines.

Nursing

There is evidence to suggest that nurses tend to see current evidence generated through nursing research as impractical and therefore irrelevant to everyday practice. Nagy et al. (2001) suggest that nurses do not see themselves as possessing sufficient skills, time or organisational support to locate, appraise and implement the best available evidence. Thompson et al. (2001) report that nurses in the UK generally do not find current guidelines, whether in printed or electronic formats, as convenient as oral information. It is likely that this is also true in Australia. Johnson and Griffiths (2001) show, however, that practice change can be promoted if practitioners are involved in processes that raise their awareness and encourage them to evaluate their own practice.

Allied health

As with any other health professions, allied health professionals have a large degree of control, autonomy and discretion over their work and are usually highly trained and skilled. The evidence-based movement poses similar issues for allied health professionals in terms of difficulty regarding environmental change where clinical knowledge, technology and professional power have been the norm for decades. Compared to medicine and nursing, however, their numbers are small and therefore their ability to generate and disseminate discipline-specific knowledge is somewhat impaired. Against this, their small numbers should make change more achievable, at least in theory.

The theory behind change

If a desired alteration in the status quo is to be achieved, then planned purposeful activity is necessary. This is in contrast to unplanned and undirected activity where the outcome is largely dependent upon chance. Planned change is 'an intended, designed, or purposeful attempt by an individual, group organisation, or larger social system to influence the status quo of itself, another organisation, or a situation' (Lippitt, 1973).

When planning change there are two major areas for consideration, namely the individuals concerned and the organisation within which the change will occur. If either is ignored, the chances of smooth progress are lessened. We generally seek to live in a state of equilibrium, and if something happens to disrupt this equilibrium, such as the acquisition of new knowledge, then an uncomfortable state of dissonance can occur where what we know does not match the way we behave.

Two courses of action can be taken. First, the new knowledge can be denied, devalued or ignored. Alternatively, there is a change in behaviour taking into account what has recently been learnt. Exactly the same principle applies in our everyday lives with such things as the use of a new piece of equipment. If time is not taken to learn how it works, and to practice handling it, then it can easily be rejected as useless, hidden at the back of a cupboard and ignored. Alternatively, the team can agree what in-service education they need to use the equipment, establish standards for safe use and put in place a plan for removal of the obsolete equipment. New knowledge can be treated in the same way.

A process for change

There are numerous models available for the transfer of evidence into clinical and professional practice, although none has been established as the 'gold standard' for implementation.

Kitson et al. (1998) suggest a multi-dimensional framework for implementing research into practice, which centres around the following concepts:

- The level and nature of the evidence
- The context or environment into which the research is to be placed
- The method or way in which the process is to be facilitated

They propose that by engaging staff members and those involved in implementing change in discussing their position on these dimensions it may be possible to devise tailored action plans that will lead to successful implementation. Of course, the strategy for change in an organisation that has poor leadership and measurement practices would be different from the strategy in an organisation that embraced a lifelong learning philosophy for all staff (Kitson et al., 1999).

Evidence suggests that successful change in health care requires an environment that is genuinely collaborative, cooperative, democratic, non-hierarchic and involves all stakeholder groups (Dowd 1994 & Martin 1997 in Dawes et al. 1999). It is proposed that involving key stakeholders will ensure a coordinated effort towards implementation and practice change that meets the requirements of all involved. This includes health care professionals, patients and relevant community interest groups, public policy makers and clinical policy makers.

Situation analysis

In order to ensure a smooth process for implementation of practice change, it is essential to assess the environment and develop an implementation plan based on findings. There are a number of elements that can support implementation. It is important to assess the structure of the organisation and the extent to which decision-making is decentralised and whether there are sufficient staff members available to support the change process. The workplace culture will impact on the success of any implementation project, and thus it is important to establish the extent to which the proposed change is consistent with the values and beliefs of the practice environment and the degree to which the culture will support change and value evidence.

Communication is another vital component, and adequate communication systems to support information exchange relating to the change and the implementation process will need to be identified. Likewise, there is a need for the identification of strong leaders who support the implementation, both visibly and behind the scenes, and they need to be engaged to support and drive the initiative. Finally, the necessary human, physical and financial resources required to support the change process should be assessed realistically with the staff who will be asked to implement the change.

Dawes et al. (1999) pose a series of questions to assist in monitoring and evaluating change. These include:

- What do you want to change?
- What do you hope to achieve by the proposed change?
- Over what time scale?
- At what cost (i.e. what resources will be involved)?
- Is there any evidence that the proposed change has worked/not worked elsewhere?
- What is the status of that evidence and what variables/measures were used in it?

- What process and outcome measures will you use to determine whether the change has been successful?
- What other aspects of practice will be affected by the proposed change (people, resources, timetabling)?
- What other people (e.g. health professionals, patients, administrators) will be affected by the proposed change, and are they cooperative?
- What are the ethical implications of introducing the proposed change (and have these been approved by the local health care ethics committees)?
- Do you have command of the necessary personnel, resources and timetabling of professional practice to introduce and maintain the proposed change?
- Is the proposed change feasible?

In practice . . .

Reflecting again on your experience of implementing change, in what ways do you recognise the aspects of the change process identified above?

When the feasibility of the implementation project has been established, it is necessary to develop a strategy for change. There are a variety of tools available to achieve this.

Tools and strategies

Education

There is hardly a better stimulus for activity than education because completion of a course requires certain activity. Education does not have to be formal to be useful. Many people have achieved much by deciding to do something informally as a group. For example, it may be feasible to have a monthly presentation of a clinical practice guideline where staff read and write or discuss ways of using that information in patient care.

Educational outreach involves face-to-face visits to the practice setting. A number of industries use this method to great effect and have influenced the actions of medical officers, pharmacists and midwives. It has been found to be cost-effective and clinically effective within local settings, used either alone or with other interventions. It is particularly effective when combined with social marketing strategies for identifying barriers to change. Social marketing is based on the view that understanding what people value can be used to motivate change.

Education should include coverage of specific behaviours to be encouraged or discouraged. It should have an understanding of motivating factors underlying current practice, and target clinicians with a high potential to become facilitators of implementation.

Continuing education, which includes credit points for professional development in recognised academic courses and other activities such as conferences, is of some benefit. However, the level of effectiveness for this strategy has not been rigorously evaluated.

Interactive education involves participation in workshops that include opportunities for discussion and participation using problem-based learning strategies. These methods are effective for addressing skill-based and knowledge-based barriers to implementation. These are the gold standard for many industries, and health is slowly catching up.

Education is likely to work most effectively when the education strategy is designed to achieve changes in actual practice. This might include, for example, learning objectives, appropriate realistic situations in which to practice learning, and feedback on practice. When health care practitioners perceive a 'compelling need' for improvement based on data in their own practice, they are more likely to feel ownership of the change process and take real steps towards achieving that change.

Decision support systems

A decision support system (DSS) is an interactive, knowledge-based computer program application that collects and presents data from a wide range of sources. It is basically a system for assisting users to make decisions based on information drawn from a wide range of sources; the information is rapidly assimilated in order to assist users to make those decisions more quickly and easily. In the case of clinical decision support systems, this definition is somewhat narrowed. A clinical decision support system (CDSS) is one that provides reminders, advice or interpretation relating to a specific client at a given time. The advice or interpretation may take the form of diagnostic assistance, critique and/or planning of therapy.

Reminders are most effective where the information is already available, and particularly where it has been incorporated into clinical information systems. Once the information is in the information systems used by health care professionals, reminders can be automated. This increases their effectiveness at changing interventions, although it is less effective for inducing changes in assessment practices.

Process-related change, or the practice of caring, and the outcomes of care interventions, can be enhanced by use of a range of devices. These include automated or manual reminders (as previously noted) and evaluation of patient and administrative systems. The benefit of using a decision support system to enhance implementation is that change can be built into the system. Context is important in health care, as is immediacy. Decision-making takes place in an instant and information is needed at the point of care at that time.

The use of automated decision support systems has been shown to facilitate change in intervention or process-based behaviour, but not in assessment or diagnostic activities. Hence use of these systems to promote assessment will be less effective than use of the systems to change specific practices. This strategy for change is most likely to be effective when the health professionals involved perceive the action required to be of benefit to patients.

Clinical audit and feedback

This strategy will be discussed in greater detail in Chapter 9. For now, it is sufficient to note that it is a continuous process that measures clinical performance and provides clinicians with an evaluation of current practice. Audit relies upon top-down support for what is essentially a bottom-up process based in the clinical setting where the measurement is to take place. It relies upon recognition that practice must change, the stimulus for which change may be a new policy, or new evidence to inform practice in the form of guidelines or evidence-based recommendations. There must also be a degree of freedom for those involved to make the necessary changes and to be provided with an opportunity to respond to feedback following evaluation.

To be effective, audit and subsequent feedback should be consistent in their key aims and objectives, and targeted to specific groups and behaviours. The methods of delivery should also be applied consistently. If used retrospectively to measure practice, the benefits of audit may be enhanced by ongoing use of reminder systems directed at sustaining either existing best practice or changed practice.

Opinion leaders

Local opinion leaders have been evaluated in a systematic review, and clinical and statistical significance was obtained in at least one outcome for each study in the review. The review concluded that opinion leaders can produce favourable results, but more research is required to identify the best context. Opinion leaders judge new information in terms of group norms, local values and realities of local practice. They make it possible for others to connect external knowledge and local context.

Local opinion leaders are not necessarily the most charismatic or authoritative figures. They are more likely to be people who are respected and sought for their clinical knowledge by their peers, who possess good listening skills and who are perceived as caring. Opinion leaders are thought to be most effective among their peers where personal knowledge has the greatest impact. Both the diffusion theory of innovation (discussed later in this chapter) and the social influence model of behaviour change rely on the use of local opinion leaders.

Recent research suggests that when best practices are clearly defined by rigorous evidence, guided quality improvement interventions using local opinion leaders can accelerate adoption of effective interventions. Such changes are especially likely 'when there is substantial room for improvements...' (Soumerai et al., 1998).

Multi-faceted approaches

Multifaceted approaches are more likely to achieve positive results as they span a number of different theoretical aspects of implementing change. A combination of two or more of the listed strategies have all been found by systematic review to be effective. In particular, health education should be considered a core activity for any combination of methods.

Audit and feedback is more effective than peer feedback in promoting change, and can lead to improved performance. This can be used to facilitate best practice implementation where the change required is intervention-based or behaviourally based, as it introduces a level of measurability not readily obtained via other methods reported in this chapter.

We have previously noted that reminders are most effective where the information is already available and particularly where it has been incorporated into clinical information systems. Once in the information systems used by health care workers, reminders can be automated. This increases their effectiveness at changing interventions but it is less effective for inducing changes in assessment practices.

Local opinion leaders can produce favourable results, but more research is required to identify the best context for using this method. This strategy is deemed to be most effective when the opinion leader's work is based on guidelines that are credible; when they recognise local circumstances and different cultures and advise practitioners on providing care in these contexts; and when practitioners see the change in practice is clear and think that it is desirable.

Marketing relates to the use of models of social influence to stimulate implementation. Again, as with interactive education, health as an industry is experiencing a delay in the uptake of new methods to sell its own message to itself. Marketing works best when combined with other strategies such as education or feedback.

Change equates to challenge. Those attempting to facilitate change have often faced significant barriers and opposition. It is essential, however, if the process is to be *meaningful* for all parties to be involved.

Decision toolkit

Decision	Tools	Evaluation
What strategy/ies should be adopted for the implementation of practice change?	Situation analysis to establish the clinical context and culture Consumer planning panel	Was the change process effective? If so, why? If not, why not?

Models for change

The transfer of evidence into practice is slow. Examples abound in medical literature of situations where research findings had a delayed entry to practice –

aspirin and thrombolytic therapy for acute MI, for instance, or anticoagulants for AF. That these interventions made it into practice at all is a chance occurrence. So, which strategies should be used? How do we design a programme? The clichéd answer is to think big, start small and act now. While no magic bullets have yet been found that will guarantee an effective change process in the health care environment, there are models available that may be of use. These are provided as examples of guides to the change process.

PDSA model

The 'plan-do-study-act' or 'PDSA' cycle is a well-used quality improvement tool. This four-phase change implementation cycle is said to assist in overcoming the natural resistance of an organisation to change. The first phase of the cycle, the 'planning' phase, involves stating the objectives of the cycle; making predictions regarding the potential outcomes and providing a rationale for those predictions; and developing a plan to implement and evaluate change that takes into account the status quo. The second phase of the cycle, the 'doing' phase, involves carrying out the plan; documenting problems encountered and observations; and starting a process of analysis and evaluation. The third, or 'study', phase involves completing the analysis, comparing data with the predictions made, and identifying potential learning objectives. The fourth phase, the 'acting' phase, involves identifying the required modifications and standardisation of new behaviours. Finally, there is the preparation of the next plan.

The cycle is implemented with continued refinement until a change that was developed within say, just one unit, is ready for broader implementation. If multiple wards used a similar approach with different interventions, the end result will be a facility with wards that have specialist knowledge on an intervention and how to implement it effectively. These wards can then be networked to facilitate broader change and overcome the natural resistance of an organisation to change.

There is much in this model that reflects the cyclical nature of action research where assessment, planning, action and reflection become the modus operandi for teams of collaborating researchers working to bring about radical change. Although theoretically promising, action research has had a chequered history in nursing and education. There have been a number of reasons for the failure of action research projects. Usually they are under-resourced, rely too heavily on one change agent and miss the fundamental importance of what Winter and Munn-Giddings (2001) describes as a 'culture of inquiry'.

Diffusion of innovation model

The diffusion of innovation model has evolved through examination of the processes by which innovations are communicated and adopted (or not). Five factors have been identified that determine the success with which an innovation or idea is adopted (Nutbeam and Harris, 1999). Understanding of these factors is central to the application of the diffusion of innovation model in the health care environment, and they are as follows:

(1) The characteristics of the potential adopters
(2) The rate of adoption
(3) The nature of the social system
(4) The characteristics of the innovations
(5) The characteristics of change agents

Diffusion of innovation theory was developed by Rogers (1983). In making the point that simply informing clinicians is insufficient to bridge the evidence gap, Sanson-Fisher (2004) explains that while research provides information on the cost-effectiveness benefit to clients of introducing a new clinical activity, that information may be less important in the adoption of the activity than the clinician's perception of whether the new activity would be advantageous. The five factors identified earlier appear to hold the key to 'relative advantage', as Rogers termed the extent to which a new activity is perceived to be better than that which it supersedes.

In practice . . .

To what extent does diffusion of innovation theory match your experience of the implementation of change?

Transtheoretical model

This model was developed in order to describe and explain different stages of change that appear to be common to most behaviour change processes. The model has two basic dimensions that describe both the different stages of change and the processes of change relevant to the different stages. The model is based on the premise that behaviour change is a process, not an event, and that individuals have varying levels of motivation or readiness to change. The process can be divided into five stages.

Stage one is concerned with what is termed 'pre-contemplation', which is when individuals are not considering the change at all. The second stage, quite appropriately termed 'contemplation', is the stage in which an individual considers making a change to a specified behaviour. This requires both knowledge and attitude change. The third and fourth stages (termed 'determination' and 'action' respectively) require a positive attitude towards change, belief in the ability to undertake change, the skill required to do so, and organisational support for change.

The final stage is 'maintenance', and relates to sustainability of the change process. This is important given that, all things being equal, there is a tendency to revert to past behaviours. Maintenance will require organisational and social support and incentive/reward systems.

Knowledge translation

Davis et al. (2003) recognise that '[a] large gulf remains between what we know and what we practice'. Furthermore they acknowledge that professional medical education and development have addressed only parts of the problem. Davis et al. (2003) propose that knowledge translation, as a holistic approach to the implementation of change, has more chance of success. They describe knowledge translation as a process that concentrates on health outcomes rather than the accrual of credits for personal promotion. It uses the local context as the place of learning and provides a range of aids or toolkits, as we have endeavoured to do in this book, to support the adoption of new knowledge. Furthermore, knowledge translation is multidisciplinary and supports the inclusion of clients and the community.

In an attempt to close the theory practice gap, Pathman et al. (1996) propose and use a two-dimensional hybrid model that requires effort from two perspectives. Their matrix for implementation presents the perspective of the target group on one axis in terms of progression through awareness, agreement and adoption to adherence and the perspective of supporters of the new knowledge. On the second axis they include considering how to predispose a target group to change by increasing knowledge; enabling the target group by promoting the best context; and reinforcing the practice once implemented.

The model is dependent on creative adoption, and a range of activities can be chosen to promote the implementation of knowledge in practice. For example, awareness may be promoted through the use of information technology, media campaigns and evidence-based practice materials; agreement is promoted through opinion leaders and small-group work; adoption may be promoted through modelling, small-group practical sessions, clinical flowcharts or academic detailing; and adherence may be promoted through reminders and audits.

In practice . . .

Consider how knowledge translation could be utilised to achieve practice change in relation to the cessation of smoking, as anticipated in the scenario described at the beginning of this chapter.

Evaluation

Evaluation of an implementation strategy endeavours to examine the structure of the programme including facilities, supplies and equipment. This includes organisational structure and the numbers and qualifications of the staff. It also seeks to analyse whether the implementation was consistent with the way the programme was planned and whether the programme can be improved. Finally, the impact of the programme is assessed in terms of whether the changes that have occurred as a result of the programme have had the desired effect.

There are a number of stages in the evaluation process. The first involves the identification of experts who will assist with the evaluation process. This may include quality assurance staff, risk management staff, epidemiologists or university staff. There may be an existing committee or individuals with experience in programme evaluation whose advice may be sought. For example, if the evaluation is concerned with infection control, the aid of an epidemiologist may be of assistance.

The second phase involves the design phase of the evaluation plan. It is recommended that the evaluation plan is kept to a simple format and includes structure, process and outcome indicators. Consider using existing data and tools. Development of new data collection tools can be very time-consuming. Using data that is already collected will give you a head start and keep costs down.

In stage three it is important to consider issues that may be faced when collecting data. This might include information such as which patients will be selected for inclusion in the programme evaluation; how feasible it is to collect data from these people in the allocated time frame; identification of the structure, process and outcome measures that you want to record; what methods are available to collect data (audits are commonly used, but other methods include questionnaires, interviews and focus group discussions); who will enter data into a computer program and who will do analysis (talk to these people before you collect any data to make sure what you want is manageable); indications of what may hinder or bias the data collection (plan a pilot study to work out feasibility issues, and check a small sample before you do any more); and who will write the report and/or present the findings (plan sufficient time for this as it almost inevitably will take longer than you anticipate).

It is essential that a realistic time frame is developed. It needs to take account of such matters as the length of time required to ensure the necessary resources are available, that data collection tools are developed or identified, the time that data collection, entry and analysis will take, and that time is available to write up and present findings.

It may also be necessary to seek approval from administrators, such as unit managers, who will need to review the evaluation plan including the objectives and outcomes. Review by administrators of other disciplines affected by the evaluation may be required, and even if it is not a requirement it may still be a good idea, as other professions may have useful suggestions.

Although programme evaluation and quality assurance may not be considered to be research as such, it may still be the case that in health care settings such activities involve ethical issues. Among those things to consider in this regard is the nature of the data to be collected. For example, collecting patient information may require ethics approval. Similarly, patient satisfaction surveys may not require a consent form but they do need an information letter, and privacy issues must be considered. Patients need to know the purpose of the survey and how their confidentiality will be preserved. Patient record numbers or names should not be used on data records; codes should be used instead.

Some organisations have an established process for the review of programmes and initiatives by patient care forums or consumers. Obtaining direct input from the people who receive the service is valuable and often provides valuable feedback.

The final phase involves preparation of the budget. This should allow for the cost of data collection, cost of analysis, and cost of evaluation and dissemination. This ensures that funds and resources (such as staff) are available.

In practice . . .

Clearly, successful change requires significant planning and organisation. Attempt to develop a plan for change in your clinical environment. Think about all of the individuals who will be affected by the change and the strategies that may help them to cope better with the change. Processes for change will vary from setting to setting, and it is important to examine the individual characteristics that are unique to your work environment and utilise approaches that are appropriate to that environment.

Conclusion

Evidence-based practice provides considerable opportunity to change professional practice and make health care more effective and efficient. No particular model is guaranteed to work, but it is essential that strategies be put in place to ensure that the specific characteristics of the individual clinical setting are accommodated.

This chapter has introduced some practical approaches to implementing evidence-based practice. This has involved an exploration of:

- Concepts fundamental to evidence-based practice
- The role of evidence-based, consensus guidelines
- The comparison of existing practice with 'best practice' through the use of clinical audit
- Ideas on the change process

In summary, to improve clinical practice we need routine mechanisms by which individuals and organisations can facilitate change. Second, while the individual's beliefs and views influence professional behaviour, so too do the organisational environment and systems in which the clinician practices. Third, choice of implementation strategy should be based on relevant research, and it should preferably involve the use of multiple, concurrent strategies. Multi-faceted approaches work more effectively than singular approaches because they address different parts of the change process. Successful practice improvement results from practice development that is adequately resourced and includes strategic partnerships to bridge institution-specific gaps in resource allocation.

Finally, any systematic approach to changing professional practice should include a plan to monitor and evaluate, and to reinforce any change. To improve clinical practice we need routine mechanisms by which individuals and organisations can facilitate change. If change is difficult to achieve, it is usually because there are some inadequacies in systems that make its achievement difficult. It does not help to target administrative practices, or some other system, and say that they prevent change, but it is useful to identify those factors within the workplace that assist the process of becoming evidence-based, and those that make it more difficult to do so.

In practice . . .

Think about the scenario presented at the beginning of this chapter and think about the extent to which the issues identified in this chapter reflect your own practice setting. Is there anything you can learn from this chapter to assist you to implement evidence-based practice in your own clinical setting? Think about what you might do in your own practice having completed this chapter, and the methods you might utilise to instigate change in the clinical environment. Now think about how you might respond to the attempts of another health professional to make changes to practice. How might you assist them in this process and provide constructive feedback through-out the change process? What do you estimate to be the chances of success?

Further reading and resources

If you are interested in learning more about the material addressed in this chapter, we would suggest the following:

Agency for Healthcare Research and Quality: www.ahrq.gov/qual/

Dunning, M., Abi-Aad, G., Gilbert, D. et al. (1997) *Turning Evidence into Everyday Practice.* London, King's Fund.

Moulding, N., Silagy, C., and Weller, D. (1999) A framework for effective management of change in clinical practice: dissemination and implementation of clinical practice guidelines. *Quality in Health Care* **8**: 177–83.

NHMRC (2000) *How to Put the Evidence into Practice: Implementation and Dissemination Strategies.* Canberra, National Health and Medical Research Council.

NHS Modernisation Agency: www.modern.nhs.uk/home/default.asp?site_id=58

National Institute of Clinical Studies: www.nicsl.com.au

Rogers, E. (1983) *Diffusion of Innovations.* New York, Free Press.

Sanson-Fisher, R.W. (2004) Diffusion of innovation theory for clinical change. *Medical Journal of Australia*, **180** (6 Suppl.): S55–S56

Winter, R. and Munn-Giddings, C. (2001) *A Handbook for Action Research in Health and Social Care.* Routledge, London.

Chapter 9

Evidence Utilisation: Clinical Audit

'Unless research-based evidence and guidance is incorporated into practice, efforts to improve the quality of care will be wasted.' – NHS CRD 1999

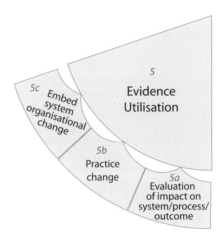

In Chapter 1 we explained the nature of evidence-based practice and the emergence and development of the evidence-based health care movement. In Chapter 2 we introduced the JBI Model of Evidence-Based Health Care and its components. In Chapter 3 we examined the nature of evidence and the various types of evidence that we consider to be useful for informing practice. In Chapter 4 we addressed the first of the substantive components of EBHC, which deals with the activity most fundamental to evidence-based practice, that is the generation of evidence. The basis of evidence-based practice is, of course, evidence. In Chapter 5 we moved on to the next component, that of the synthesis of evidence, and began to take you through the process of the systematic review. In so doing, we dealt only with the first half of the systematic review, locating the evidence. The second half of the systematic review process – the appraisal and evaluation of the evidence – we addressed in Chapter 6 where we took you through the processes and issues associated with the synthesis of different forms of evidence. In Chapter 7 we dealt with the transfer of evidence including the report of the systematic review and the development of clinical guidelines. In Chapter 8, the process of getting evidence into practice – the broad rubric of evidence utilisation – was addressed with an emphasis on the use of clinical guidelines.

Now we arrive at the final component on the dial of the clock in the JBI Model. This component, and thus this chapter, addresses the utilisation of evidence. Here we continue to examine the ways in which evidence can be incorporated into practice. We introduced the concept of clinical audit in Chapter 8, but here we examine this mechanism in detail. Clinical audit is a strategy in which health care practitioners at every level of their career can be involved. Audits can both affirm practice and point to areas in need of closer alignment with contemporary evidence, and in this chapter we explain how the process of clinical audit can assist in the process of getting evidence into practice.

This chapter focuses on the clinical audit and feedback process as a method of promoting evidence utilisation and discusses:

- Clinical audit
- The steps in clinical audit
- Systems to support a clinical audit and feedback programme

In practice . . .

A friend of yours has attempted to quit smoking on several occasions during the time you have known each other. However, he is already overweight and every time he quits smoking he ends up even heavier because he refuses to exercise and substitutes the cigarettes with food. You have told him about the guidelines you were involved in developing at work and he asks if they have been successful. The guidelines developed regarding smoking cessation were finally accepted and successfully implemented, but how do you assess whether there has been an improvement in either organisational or patient outcomes?

As you read through this chapter, keep in mind your friend's situation. At various points you will be asked to think about how the content might relate to this case and whether it offers any solutions or strategies for assisting him.

Introduction

The systematic and critical analysis of the quality of clinical care is of significant importance. The evidence on the effectiveness of strategies to facilitate the transfer of research-based recommendations into practice is limited. Numerous systematic reviews have focused on specific approaches, strategies and interventions, but there is no strong evidence to support any single approach. A systematic review reported by the Centre for Reviews and Dissemination (1999) suggests that multiple interventions seem to be more effective than single interventions, but they conclude that implementation is a difficult and complex process. They go on to suggest that improving clinical effectiveness in health care requires the establishment of 'routine mechanisms by which individual and organisational change can occur'.

They state that evidence indicates a need for steps to be pursued in programmes designed to transfer and utilise evidence, including 'a diagnostic analysis to identify factors likely to influence the proposed change, and a choice of dissemination and implementation interventions should be guided by the diagnostic analysis and informed by knowledge and relevant research'.

They point out that 'multi-faceted interventions targeting different barriers to change are more likely to be effective than single interventions' and that 'any systematic approach to changing professional practice should include plans to monitor and evaluate and maintain and reinforce any change'.

Of those strategies found to be moderately effective, audit and feedback appear to be the most promising. Educational outreach in the form of academic detailing appears to have some positive effect in the area of prescribing, but continuing education and the dissemination of evidence summaries do not appear to impact on implementation. Clinical audit provides an opportunity to monitor practice where changes to care delivery have been introduced and to ascertain whether the change to an intervention has had a positive and effective impact on health outcomes. This chapter will endeavour to provide readers with a comprehensive examination of the three stages of the clinical audit process and provide some strategies to promote successful auditing. An explanation of clinical effectiveness is provided first, for the sake of clarity.

Clinical effectiveness

Clinical effectiveness is the extent to which clinical interventions, when administered to a specific patient population, achieve the intended effect. It is about doing the right thing, in the right way, for the right patient (NHS Executive, 1998). Clinical effectiveness is an umbrella term for a range of activities that are concerned with achieving quality patient care based on the best available evidence. It includes best-practice-focused activities such as systematic reviews, clinical guidelines and clinical audit (Dickinson, 1998).

The three components to achieving clinical effectiveness are:

- *Informing:* ensuring practitioners, patients and managers know what interventions are clinically effective based on the best available evidence.
- *Changing:* using this knowledge to review current patient care and to apply effective practice within the clinical setting.

Consumers are becoming increasingly interested in clinical effectiveness as they become more informed, have greater expectations and are more involved in decision-making (Dickinson, 1998).

Clinical audit

Clinical audit is a tool that addresses all the components of clinical effectiveness in the ongoing goal of improving the quality of health care. Clinical audit is a process that health professionals use to examine their care practices and compare the results with clinical guidelines or best practice statements (Kinn, 1995). Clinical audit is best considered as an internal mechanism for health professionals to use for quality improvement.

The process of clinical audit provides a systematic framework for establishing care standards based on best evidence, and comparing day-to-day practice to these standards. By conducting clinical audits, health professionals can identify areas of care that require improvement and/or change; or can provide evidence that the care currently being provided is of a high quality (Burnett and Winyard, 1998).

Like clinical effectiveness, the primary goals of clinical audit are improving patient care, improving health outcomes and effectively translating research into practice. Clinical audit is not a process through which the most effective care practices are established – this is the role of research. Clinical audit, however, does provide a bridge between research and practice by comparing the two, identifying any inconsistencies and developing action plans for improvement. The processes incorporated in a clinical audit address this major challenge of moving research-derived knowledge into the practice setting.

The steps of clinical audit offer a framework to establish clinical guidelines (*inform*); assess current practice and implement changes (*change*) and monitor the effects (*monitor*). It therefore provides a vital link in evidence-based practice (Garland and Corfield, 1999).

Morrell and Harvey (1999) introduce the ideas behind clinical audit. You will notice that, like much of the literature in this subject, the content is quite UK-specific, as clinical audit is widely used in the UK. However, the general principles are of broader application.

Benefits of clinical audit

Many health professionals see clinical audit as a practical means of translating guidelines into practice change, improving quality, and maintaining professional standards. The framework of clinical effectiveness and clinical audit offers benefits for all stakeholders in health care. The stakeholders and identified benefits are as follows.

Patients: The main focus of clinical effectiveness should be achieving a quality outcome for the patient including:

- Consistent care with less individual practitioner variation
- Timely management of health problems
- Improved information and education about care

Nurses and other health professionals: Involvement in clinical auditing and a system of promoting clinically effective care can lead to:

- Greater understanding of evidence-based practice
- The ability to achieve and maintain professional credibility
- Decision-making and actions being able to be justified on a scientific rather than an intuitive basis
- Experience in designing and carrying out research and quality improvement projects

- Improved job satisfaction as professional skills are used in the most effective way
- Increased communication and teamwork

Managers: Support of clinical effectiveness and use of clinical audit can offer:

- Quality care that is the focus of accreditation
- Demonstrable attainment of care standards
- Identification of good practice as well as areas for improvement
- Decision making and policy generation on a scientific rather than an intuitive base
- Consistent decision-making by clinicians that leads to reduced variation in the provision of care and which can be more cost-effective

Government/funding bodies of health care: Clinical effectiveness has much to offer governments and funding bodies of health care including:

- Reduced variability in care practices between individual health care facilities (this does not mean reduction in individualised care, but rather cessation of practices not supported by best evidence)
- Maximising cost effectiveness
- Increased consumer satisfaction

In practice . . .

In what ways is clinical audit currently used in your workplace? How does it impact upon your professional practice? What is the attitude of clinicians to this mechanism for the translation of evidence into practice?

The clinical audit process

Clinical audit is described as a cyclic process, incorporating systematic steps to work through the cycle (Figure 9.1).

The key stages of clinical audit are:

- Determining an audit topic and defining agreed standards of care
- Collecting data on current practice
- Evaluating the findings to identify any required improvements and/or to highlight quality practice
- Acting to implement change
- Re-evaluation of practice through repeating the audit steps

Planning a clinical audit

Before commencing a clinical audit it is important to have a formal project plan identifying the objective of the clinical audit, how it will be conducted, who will be involved, and a time frame for completion. An auditor must be clear on what

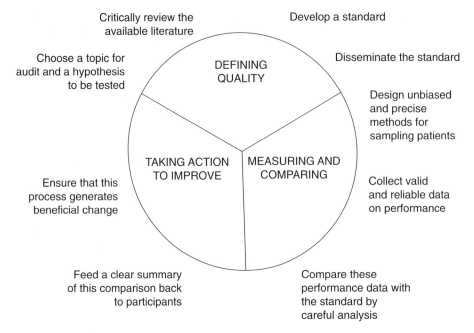

Fig. 9.1 The audit cycle (adapted from Morgan and Fennessy, 1996).

questions are being asked and how the information will be gathered to provide the answers.

Stage one: defining best practice

The major steps in this stage are as follows.

(1) Choosing a topic: Note that the goal of clinical effectiveness – achieving the best outcome for the patient – should be kept in mind when selecting an audit topic. Health practitioners, managers and patients should all be involved in the selection of audit topics in areas where significant improvements to the clinical care can be made. There should be feasible ways to make improvements or changes to the area of care if the clinical audit is going to be of any benefit, although it should be kept in mind that raising awareness of an issue is the first step to change.

Factors to consider when prioritising topics for clinical auditing include:

- Has the issue been identified by stakeholders as a concern (e.g. patient complaints)?
- Is there a wide variation in current practice (e.g. many nurses do it differently)?
- Is it an area of high risk (e.g. high level of morbidity and/or mortality)?
- Is it an area of high volume (e.g. is it something that is done regularly)?
- Is it an area of high cost (e.g. will you be able to reduce or justify the cost)?

- Is there access to the required internal and external resources (e.g. time, information, staff)? (Burnett and Winyard, 1998; Morrell and Harvey, 1999)

(2) Defining best practice – clinical guidelines and audit indicators: After the topic for auditing has been clearly stated, a guideline (care standard) should be developed setting out what best practice is and how it is to be achieved. Care standards should be based on evidence that they are clinically effective, and should be relevant to the local patient population and facility.

To develop appropriate clinical guidelines, a review of best evidence should be undertaken to determine the most clinically effective care. As you will have noted in previous chapters, performing a complete review of best evidence to develop care standards is an arduous task, so auditors may choose to utilise pre-existing clinical guidelines to develop care standards. Clinical or best practice guidelines are systematically developed statements based on best evidence that assist clinicians to make decisions about appropriate resident care. Often, national bodies (e.g. Joanna Briggs Institute; Royal College of Nursing Australia) develop and disseminate broad clinical guidelines based on systematic research reviews. Adapting existing clinical guidelines into locally appropriate care standards ensures that the defined standard of care is based on sound evidence, and is a good starting point for auditors lacking time and/or resources to conduct complete systematic reviews (Morrell and Harvey, 1999).

In developing or adapting care standards, auditors should ensure that the resulting care standards are:

- Relevant to local stakeholders (patients, staff, managers, health care facility)
- Based on clear evidence
- Reliable (different practitioners will be able to interpret and apply them in the same way)
- Valid (the objective of care will be achieved if the standard is adhered to)
- Flexible and reviewable (Burnett and Winyard, 1998)

The clinical guideline identified for the audit topic will be used retrospectively during the clinical audit to assess the quality of the practice that occurred. To use clinical guidelines to assess practice they need to be developed into quantitative criteria, or 'indicators'. Indicators are:

'Quantitative statements, which are used to measure quality of care. Indicators always include a percentage, ratio or other quantitative way of saying how many patients/clients the expected care should be provided for.'
(National Centre for Clinical Audit, 1997)

The following example demonstrates how an indicator might be developed.

Clinical guideline: A fluid intake sheet is the best method of monitoring daily fluid intake (Joanna Briggs Institute (2001) Maintaining Oral Hydration in Older People, Best Practice 5(1))

Indicator: 100% of patients on fluid monitoring will have a fluid intake sheet completed on a daily basis

The indicators you develop must be measurable, observable and relate to only one specific area of practice. Indicators should be focused on:

> *'the goal of achieving the best outcome for residents. This will ensure that you have a clear means of evaluating whether the day-to-day practice you observe is meeting the care standards.'* (Garland and Corfield, 1999)

(3) Dissemination: After the audit team has developed the care standard and audit indicators, the expected standard of care needs to be distributed to all stakeholders. Practitioners, managers and patients should know the expected outcomes of interventions that are initiated and how they can most effectively achieve the outcomes.

Sharing the standards of best practice allows those who will be affected by them to give some input or feedback to the audit team. As we have noted in earlier chapters, for effective implementation of any change in practice it is important that staff members feel a 'sense of ownership'. Exchanging information and being open to feedback from colleagues will raise awareness of your audit activity, encourage communication and improve the adoption rate of new practice guidelines.

Disseminating your care standards can be as simple as circulating your proposed document, using notice boards or sharing at staff meetings or hand-over.

Stage two: measurement and comparison

You will note from this chapter that the auditor should look closely at each audit indicator and decide how data will be collected to determine whether the standard has been met. It is helpful to identify criteria that need to be met to achieve the standard.

'Structure criteria' are the resources, or what is needed to implement the standard – knowledge, staff, time, equipment, and organisational structure.

'Process criteria' refers to what needs to be done to implement the care standard – the actions to take and the decisions to make. The process will include aspects such as assessment, evaluation, referral, documentation and specific practical interventions.

'Outcome criteria' are the anticipated results of the intervention, or what you are expecting to achieve through implementing the care standard (Morrell and Harvey, 1999; Kinn, 1995).

For example, let's assume that your pain management audit has been designed to investigate the care standard 'all patients will have a pain assessment documented on admission'. The audit team establishes that the two indicators for this standard are '100% of patients will be assessed for the presence of pain on the day of admission' and '100% of patients will have their pain assessment documented in their history'.

What structure criteria need to be in place for this to occur? Consider the following possible criteria:

- The admitting nurse is competent in pain assessment.
- There is a practice and policy manual to inform staff, which is informed by evidence-based requirements for pain assessment.
- There is time and an appropriate area in which to perform an assessment.
- There is a system of documentation.

What are the process criteria that need to occur for this indicator to be met? Consider the following possible criteria:

- The nurse implements policies and procedures as defined.
- The nurse initiates discussions with patients regarding pain.
- The nurse assesses for presence of pain.
- The nurse documents and communicates the patient's pain status.

What are the outcome criteria? Consider the following possible criteria:

- All patients have been assessed for pain in accordance with the practice and policy manual.
- All patients' pain assessments have been recorded.
- All patients' pain levels are documented and communicated.

It is useful to gather data from a variety of sources such as patient histories/documentation and patients themselves to ensure the capture of all possible information that will help decide if the care standard has been met. The audit should be designed so that data is collected on as many criteria as possible, as this will provide a sound base on which to make decisions for implementing change in the next audit step. Data collection tools such as checklists or questionnaires can be designed specifically for the audit or can be adapted from pre-existing collection tools. When collecting and recording the data, the auditor should be considerate of basic research principles such as ethical considerations and confidentiality. The audit team may need to select an audit sample. It may not be possible to review the care of every person in your facility. The sample size, however, should be large enough to give an overall representation of the practice within your facility.

Collecting data is the most visible part of the audit process and may include record reviews, checklists, questionnaires, interview or observation. While some people argue that it is better to have someone new to the area who has no preconceived ideas or prejudices that will affect his or her observation of practice, it is usually acceptable to have a qualified clinician auditing patient care. The auditor needs to have an understanding of the clinical process, the interventions that she or he is observing and the documentation, as clinical audit is a method for health professionals to assess their own clinical care. Thus, it is appropriate for clinicians to collect the objective data.

Evaluating the data involves comparing the findings on day-to-day practice with the care standards outlining expected practice. To do this, actual findings are compared to the quantitative indicators that were developed during the first stage of audit.

Where the standards of practice have not been met, a thorough audit will look at *why* best practice has not occurred. Understanding why the day-to-day practice that was observed did not meet the care standards is important for the next stage of audit – developing an action plan. Using multiple data collection techniques that look at the structures, processes and outcomes will help establish the cause of the problem.

For example, let's assume that you use a checklist to collect information on smoking cessation and review the patients' histories for evidence. You find that there are no notes regarding advice on smoking cessation. With the information you have, can you establish whether advice was provided on smoking cessation? How will you know what to do to improve practice?

However, consider an alternative strategy. You use a simple checklist, staff questionnaire and interview patients to determine if smoking cessation information is being provided. When you review the patient histories you find no evidence of smoking cessation advice documented. However, when you interview patients you establish that nursing staff ask them about their smoking experiences and initiate smoking cessation techniques as required, and patients state that they are generally smoke-free. Your questionnaire results indicate that nursing staff are very knowledgeable about providing smoking cessation advice. It is also an indicator that many staff are unaware of the procedures for documenting the provision of such advice, and some staff answer that they do not have time to write a full assessment in the history when the patient is admitted. With the information you have gathered from multiple sources and using a variety of data collection techniques, you have greater insight into practice and possible strategies that you might use to implement improvements.

Your analysis might find that care practices did meet the standards that were defined from best evidence and that the outcomes of care are being achieved in the most effective manner. It is important to feed this finding back to the stakeholders.

Stage three: acting to achieve change

As you can see, once the audit results have been analysed and the audit team have identified reasons why the practice has fallen short of the standard, it is time to develop a plan for improvement. In developing an action plan the audit team should identify:

- An appropriate course of action for improvement
- Who is responsible for initiating each step of the course of action
- A time frame for completing the action plan
- A time frame for re-auditing to evaluate change in practice

For example, let us assume that in your smoking cessation audit you determined that patients were being provided with advice on smoking cessation on admission but there were barriers to nursing staff meeting the second indicator. The care standard was therefore not met. The collected data indicated that it was structure criteria that prevented the standard being met: lack of time to document, and lack of knowledge about the requirements of documentation.

To implement change you would need to address both of these structure criteria. First, it would be necessary to modify the system. This might involve the development of a streamlined documentation system that could include, for example, an easy-to-complete smoking cessation chart. Second, it would be necessary to attend to the relevant education deficits of the staff, and in the present example that would mean ensuring that nursing staff had received training on documentation skills.

Deciding on an appropriate action plan may seem like a challenge, but often after comparing the audit data to the care standard statement it is clear what changes need to be made to meet best practice. At this point the audit team need to brainstorm various solutions to the problem to come up with a plan of action that will achieve the desired outcome – clinical effectiveness.

In considering how to go about change, it is helpful to think about areas that may need to be addressed to achieve clinical effectiveness.

Education: Education will only be beneficial in achieving changed practice where a lack of knowledge was identified as a major reason for poor practice. Education strategies include one-to-one exchange of information; seminars and workshops; access to literature; and notice board displays.

Changing the system: When the audit has identified problems with access to supplies, systems of documentation, staff skills mix, work load, and so forth, the audit team will need to develop strategies to change the system. Strategies might include changing the filing system, increasing staffing numbers or skills mix, or increasing access to resources.

Changing behaviour: Where the audit has identified staff performance as the reason for failure to meet best practice, the audit team must carefully assess the reasons. If it is clear that resources are available and staff members have the knowledge and skills to perform the care according to best practice, then strategies to address poor performance need to be identified.

Re-auditing: After the action plan has been implemented, the audit cycle continues to the evaluation phase. It is necessary to re-audit to determine whether the actions have been successful in improving practice. Re-auditing will either demonstrate improvements in practice or indicate that there are still improvements to be made to reach best practice standards.

Remember – stakeholders like to hear about successes too! Feeding back positive results to managers, staff and patients highlights good practice and the quality of the care the facility provides, and gives everyone reason to be proud of the achievement. It also inspires the team to start working on a new audit topic!

Strategies to promote successful auditing

The ultimate success of auditing in achieving best practice depends on the implementation strategy within the facility, and the structures in place to support the auditing process. Managerial support is the key factor in facilitating a successful audit because without a coordinated approach, integration with other quality improvement activities, and access to resources, clinical auditing will not of itself bring about positive results (Johnston et al., 2000). Other factors that will impact upon the success of clinical auditing include the following.

Teamwork: Establishing a team of multidisciplinary health clinicians who will be able to communicate and plan with each other will bring a variety of experiences, skills and ideas to the audit, ensuring that the process meets the needs of all key stakeholders.

Training: It is helpful to have at least some members of the audit team trained in audit skills and experienced in designing and implementing projects.

Dedicated time: It is important to remember that clinical auditing takes time! Without dedicated time to be involved in audit activity staff members will be overloaded and care standards may decline.

Access to information: Clinical auditors will require access to best evidence (e.g. through journal subscription, links to professional groups, access to databases). Access to internal information such as resident histories will also be essential to conducting audit.

Communication: Keeping everyone informed of the process and maintaining an awareness of the overall aims of the audit will increase input from staff and encourage uptake of practice changes. Good communication will also decrease the possibility of staff feeling threatened because they are ill-informed.

Patient involvement: Achieving the best possible outcome for patients is the primary focus of clinical auditing. Involving patients as much as possible can increase the success of the audit in meeting the primary objective. Patients could be involved on the audit team; patient feedback could be considered when determining audit topics, and talking to patients during the audit process to determine their perception of the area of audit are all ways to ensure that patients are involved (Johnston et al., 2000; Morrell and Harvey, 1999).

Writing an audit report

When the audit is completed a report should be written to inform all the stakeholders of the results. Audit reports also provide a record of your continuous improvement activities for quality improvement processes such as accreditation.

A report should outline the whole process clearly. It would commence with a description of the background of your audit – your audit topic, why you decided on the topic, costs of the audit, and a brief description of the participants/ auditors and how they were involved in the process. You should also identify any input from other stakeholders in the audit (e.g. feedback from patients or staff).

The report should include the guidelines that were used to assess clinical practice, and the sources used to develop the guidelines (e.g. systematic reviews, JBI Best Practice Information Sheets, national clinical guidelines).

The method used to conduct the audit should be described, including what aspects of practice were being audited, who conducted the auditing, what methods were used, the data that was collected in the audit and how this was analysed.

The findings should be set out clearly and the conclusions drawn from the findings should be explained. Any process of peer reviewing would also be outlined to give strength to the conclusions. A statement identifying clearly whether the objectives were achieved or not should be included.

The report would go on to outline the improvements that were planned to address areas of practice that did not meet the indicators defined in the audit. You might include what practice you changed and how, the rationale for the action plan, who was involved, how you went about changing practice and any problems you encountered.

If there is evidence already of improved practice, include this in your report. If you are yet to reassess clinical practice following implementation of the action plan, include in your report when you will be re-auditing, and any other follow-ups that are required following the audit, including any recommendations made by the audit team.

The best practice model would not be complete without a process of evaluating whether change has been successful and resulted in improved outcomes for professionals and patients and a *meaningful* journey for all involved.

Decision toolkit

Decision	Tools	Evaluation
How to assess organisational and patient outcomes?	A process for clinical audit.	Was there any improvement in practice? Was best practice already in place?

Practical tools for clinical audit

Evidence transfer remains one of the biggest challenges facing the evidence-based practice movement in health care. It often requires investment at both the organisational and practitioner levels and the use of multiple strategies and interventions. Essentially, implementing evidence represents the age-old problem of health care: how to manage change. There will never be an easy one-size-fits-all solution to this ongoing problem associated with changing practice and the way people feel about change. However, a variety of programmes have been developed in recent years to assist with the clinical audit process. Probably the two most recent include Audit-maker (Flinders University) and PACES (the Joanna Briggs Institute).

Audit-maker

The Australian Centre for Evidence-based Clinical Practice has developed a clinical audit tool, aptly named Audit-maker. This tool has been developed in order to assist clinicians to set up a clinical audit database.

Built on an ACCESS® platform, the first few screens of this tool are designed to help you clarify exactly what type of audit you want to do. To begin with, you are prompted to enter a title for your audit and then to choose whether it is retrospective, prospective or both. If this kind of terminology is enough to frighten you off, don't despair. Simply click on the help menu and the prompts will help you determine what type of audit you are going to do. Then the tool asks you to identify what the goals of your audit are and what outcomes you are interested in. By the time you have filled out the first half-dozen responses, you can generate a draft/outline for your ethics proposal by simply clicking a button.

The data entry screens are similarly easy to establish. They include in-built demographic and co-morbidity menus as well as the ability to add your own personal choices. The tool also has a series of standard reports that can be printed out, which summarise the data that has been entered to date. So you do not have to wait for six or twelve months to get a statistician to analyse your data – you can look at simple summaries (including means and medians) at the click of a button. For those of you wanting a more sophisticated analysis, the information in your database can be exported, at any stage, to EXCEL® and then to a package such as SPSS® for further manipulation.

PACES

The Practical Application of Clinical Evidence System (PACES) is an audit-based program developed by the Joanna Briggs Institute. It is designed to meet the specific needs of both clinicians and quality improvement staff in health care organisations. This program strongly compliments the Audit-maker program. Paces, however, differs from Audit-maker in a number of important respects. The PACES program is web-based and has defined audit indicators upon which to base the audit. The audit indicators have been derived from best available evidence and are used for benchmarking within the quality improvement style audits. For benchmarking to occur, it is essential that the same audit indicators are used. The program involves the collection of data relevant to a specific topic. Thus, using pre-determined audit indicators, baseline data is collected either manually or from a printout, or by using a specially designed hand-held computer. This data is then fed back into the PACES program for evaluation, report and feedback.

GRIP

GRIP is an acronym for 'Getting Research Into Practice'. This module was developed to establish inter-professional processes within teams to identify and examine barriers to the utilisation of evidence, and design implementation programs to overcome the barriers identified. If an audit shows a less than perfect compliance with the indicators, the online generic work plan (GRIP) assists the user in problem-identification, action-planning and action-taking to improve compliance with the audit indicators, prior to commencing a follow-up, post-action audit.

The audit team then has the opportunity to compare the pre-action/intervention results. This process can be repeated until the team is content with the results. Also available is an on-line facility to submit data to the Joanna Briggs Institute for benchmarking with other 'like' organisations.

Clinical audit and research

There has been some debate over the years as to whether clinical audit constitutes a form of clinical research. Regardless of which argument you favour, both play an important and often complementary role in improving clinical practice. One argument is that research utilises methods that extend knowledge and that clinical audit is merely an assessment of whether clinical practice is in line with the research evidence. However, similarities should be acknowledged, with both processes engaging in a process of enquiry and both gathering and analysing information, and with many drawing similarities between clinical audit and action research. Morrell and Harvey (1999) identify four links between clinical audit and research.

(1) Research informs the clinical audit process by providing the evidence for standards and criteria against which practice is measured.
(2) Clinical audit informs researchers of where the results of audit provoke new research questions.
(3) Research methods (such as literature review, data collection and data analysis) are applied to the design of a clinical audit.
(4) Research is used to evaluate the effectiveness of clinical audit so that the process of audit itself is examined and evaluated.

It could also be argued that clinical audit does in fact have the potential to create new knowledge as an assessment tool for the effectiveness of various implementation strategies. In this sense clinical audit can in fact directly inform clinical practice with regard to implementation.

Conclusion

Undertaking a clinical audit can result in numerous benefits to clinical practice, and governments, health services and health professional organisations are now acknowledging the importance of investing in the development and evaluation of utilisation methodologies. This is supported by the development of utilisation initiatives by the National Institute of Health and Clinical Excellence in England, the Agency for Healthcare Research and Quality in the United States and the National Institute for Clinical Studies in Australia. These agencies are pursuing a range of initiatives to promote evidence utilisation and/or engage in primary research designed to evaluate the efficacy or otherwise of utilisation approaches.

Significant benefits of the clinical audit process include:

- The promotion of reflection on the quality of the clinical care delivered
- Developments in team-building and collaboration
- The implementation of changes in clinical practice and improvements in patient experiences and patient outcomes

This chapter has provided a framework and established processes for the conduct of clinical audit. With the development of new resources to assist with the process of clinical audit, such as Audit-maker and PACES, processes will become more streamlined and less time-consuming.

In practice . . .

It is almost guaranteed that at some point in your career you will experience, or be involved in some way in, a clinical audit of practice. Just as the organisation for which you work has a responsibility to establish strategies and systems to ensure that practice is of the highest level, so too do you as a health professional have a responsibility to be committed to a culture of clinical excellence in practice.

Being involved in a clinical audit provides you with an opportunity to enhance your professional development, to work and learn as part of a multidisciplinary team and to reflect upon your practice. Think about what your personal learning objectives are and how being involved in the clinical audit process might assist you in achieving those goals.

You should now be in a position to respond to your friend's question as to whether the guidelines for cessation of smoking have been successful.

Further reading and resources

If you are interested in learning more about the material addressed in this chapter, we would suggest the following:

Audit-maker is available for downloading from the Australian Centre for Evidence-Based Clinical Practice website: www.acebcp.org.au

PACES is available to corporate members of the Joanna Briggs Institute via their website: www.joannabriggs.edu.au

Burnett, A. and Winyard, G. (1998) Clinical audit at the heart of clinical effectiveness. *Journal of Quality in Clinical Practice* **18** (1): 3–19.

Joanna Briggs Institute (2001) *Acute Care Clinical Auditing Manual*. JBI, Adelaide.

Morgan, L. and Fennessy, G. (1996) How to undertake clinical audit: a new service. *Nursing Standard* **10** (5): 32–3.

Morrell, C. and Harvey, G. (1999) *The Clinical Audit Handbook: Improving the Quality of Health Care*. London, Baillière Tindall.

National Institute for Health and Clinical Excellence (NICE) (2002) *Principles for Best Practice in Clinical Audit*

Chapter 10

Evidence-Based Practice: Issues and Challenges

'The best thing about the future is that it only comes one day at a time.' – Abraham Lincoln

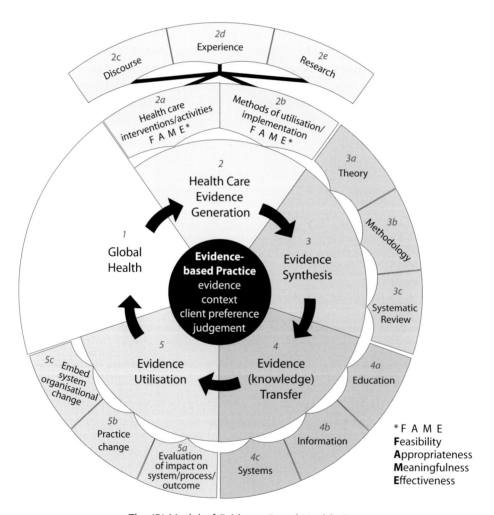

The JBI Model of Evidence-Based Health Care

Now we have come full circle on the clock dial of the JBI Model. In Chapter 1 we explained the nature of evidence-based practice and the emergence and development of the evidence-based health care movement. In Chapter 2 we introduced the JBI Model of Evidence-Based Health Care and its components. In Chapter 3 we examined the nature of evidence and the various types of evidence that we consider to be useful for informing practice. In Chapter 4 we addressed the first of the substantive components of EBHC which deals with the activity most fundamental to evidence-based practice, that is the generation of evidence. In Chapter 5 we moved on to the synthesis of evidence and began to take you through the process of the systematic review. In so doing, we dealt only with the first half of the systematic review, locating the evidence. Appraisal and evaluation of the evidence we addressed in Chapter 6 where we took you through the processes and issues associated with the synthesis of different forms of evidence. In Chapter 7 we dealt with the transfer of evidence including the report of the systematic review and the development of clinical guidelines. In Chapter 8, evidence utilisation was addressed with an emphasis on the use of clinical guidelines. In Chapter 9 we explained the process of clinical audit and how it can assist in the process of getting evidence into practice. This final chapter contextualises EBHC amid contemporary issues and challenges. Here we discuss diverse and pertinent issues including the organisational context of health care, legal and policy considerations, the appropriate place for clinical guidelines in professional practice, the role of consumers, and the information explosion along with its associated technology.

This chapter discusses the promotion of global health through basing practice on the evidence in relation to:

- Health care organisations
- Legal frameworks
- Future trends
- Information technology

In practice . . .

Today, more than ever, health professionals must consider not only the anatomical or physiological viewpoint of the clinical care they provide, but also the legal, ethical, and social issues associated with that care. You are discussing these issues with a friend of yours who is a teacher and he indeed sympathises with your situation. More and more, in all industries, there is a reliance on evidence to support practice and avoid potential litigation. To add to the frustrations of achieving this in a global community where information generation is forever increasing, professionals have to find rigorous and reliable ways of reviewing that evidence.

As you read through this chapter, keep in mind your friend's situation. At various points you will be asked to think about how the content might relate to this case and whether it offers any solutions or strategies for assisting him.

Introduction

Evidence-based practice has made significant progress since its inception. Initiatives that endeavour to embed evidence in practice have continued to break new ground with regard to the inclusion of broader definitions of evidence and the implementation of clinical practice guidelines. There is much to consider when envisioning the future of evidence-based practice and its broader implications.

Legal regulation of the principles of health care intervention and the organisation of medical services is an increasingly important field. To establish a case of medical negligence, a plaintiff must prove on the balance of probabilities that the defendant has acted in breach of a duty of care that was owed to the injured plaintiff. A major hurdle for any medical negligence claim is the requirement of proof that the injury was caused by medical negligence, particularly in areas where there is considerable uncertainty surrounding the nature of a condition or where there may be other possible factors that trigger a disease.

This chapter considers future directions for the evidence-based movement. It will examine the current status and trends of the evidence-based movement from both an individual and an organisational perspective; guideline development and utilisation; and legal implications.

Evidence-based practice and the role of organisations

Health professionals need to understand the organisational context and its requirements if evidence-based practice is to evolve in a palatable and viable form. The boundaries of health care are changing and it is important to understand how it is transforming. It is also important to appreciate the role that evidence-based practice is playing in that change. Knowledge management has emerged as a significant factor in the delivery of health care and as such, the introduction of evidence-based decision-making into an organisation may require substantial modification of the organisational culture. The establishment of a culture of evidence-based practice necessitates a particular emphasis on learning, and if that is absent, it must be developed. This is consistent with contemporary thinking around the notion of lifelong learning but it nevertheless requires a concerted effort to inculcate such a culture among health professionals who already feel overtaxed by their clinical responsibilities.

The organisational context

Muir-Gray (2001) is very much concerned with a manager's perspective, arguing that the parameters used as a basis for decision-making about resource allocation have changed as a result of the evolution of evidence-based health care and the development of a new management agenda. Muir-Gray (2001) states that until now the evolution of clinical practice has been fragmented, uncoordinated, and driven by individual clinicians, which is unacceptable. It is argued that those responsible for management and funding of health services must develop a new consultative relationship in which clinicians and managers can work together to guide the course of the evolution of clinical practice.

Other writers have also examined the organisational context of evidence-based practice. For example, Mitchell (1998) conducted a case study to examine the organisational factors that promote, sustain or inhibit evidence-based practice. The study suggested that improvements in information management were necessary, not only for health professionals but also to enhance the knowledge and choice for patients in relation to their care. This is congruent not only with the philosophy of evidence-based practice but, more fundamentally, with 'consumerism' in health care. Power and clinical autonomy are sensitive issues, but this study identified strategies to 'de-personalise' the debate on evidence-based practice. Mitchell (1998) suggests that moving the debate from individual to organisational concerns is more likely to prove a successful strategy in achieving change.

Much has been said (and written) about the role of the organisation. In particular, the discussion has emphasised the place of power and the potential for evidence-based guidelines to be used as a tool for shaping practice. Much has also been said of the need to involve professional groups in the development of an evidence-based practice culture within an organisation. This is a prerequisite for success in such an endeavour.

Kenrick and Luker (1996) further develop the theme of the place of management in research utilisation, but do so in the context of a district nursing service. Their focus is on the utilisation of research by district nurses who deliver their services in a professionally insular setting, usually isolated from any form of peer review. Their perspective is that of a manager of a district nursing service faced with the ever-increasing imperative to deliver high-quality, effective and efficient services. The authors investigated the link between management culture and clinical practice in an attempt to gain insights that would assist in this task.

Apart from providing an interesting profile of a group of nurse managers, Kenrick and Luker conclude that effective, evidence-based practice depends on having a positive organisational culture. An interesting point about this study is the extent to which their own practice is evidence-based. There is an ambiguous allusion to this when they discuss the managers' practices and the extent to which their own practices are evidence-based. It is not altogether clear whether they are referring to the managers' clinical practices or managerial practices. However, if the managerial practices are evidence-based, the question remains as to the quality of the evidence. Health professions do not have a monopoly on either evidence-based practice or poor-quality research.

In practice . . .

Your friend the teacher will no doubt have a strong interest in the foregoing material. How do you see the principles of evidence-based practice translating into a profession such as teaching, or put another way, a discipline such as education?

A powerful source of motivation for governments and organisations to work towards evidence-based health care is the desire to extract the maximum benefit from every dollar expended on health. Apart from the constant pressure to increase the amount spent by government on health care, there is a growing recognition that money spent has not always been spent wisely. In the past, most of the health dollar has been spent under the direction of medical practitioners alone. Every nurse has a repertoire of anecdotes about the purchase of million-dollar medical equipment while they struggle to acquire the most basic equipment for their ward. Muir-Gray has a number of comments on the relationship between evidence-based health care and the pragmatics of expenditure and purchasing.

In essence, Muir-Gray points to the purchasing being determined by those who hold power, rather than according to pragmatic need. This is not new but it does highlight the lack of logic and rationality in this approach. If health professionals in all disciplines practice on the basis of evidence (and purchasing reflects this practice), then it is reasonable to assume that the benefit will be maximised for every dollar spent. This is as true for nurses as for medical practitioners, although the amounts involved may differ considerably. Health services have the opportunity to make substantial savings by adopting an appropriate purchasing philosophy.

In practice . . .

How closely allied are evidence-based practice and economic rationalism? It is sometimes argued that the former is very much a creature of the latter. Is the one symptomatic of the other?

Legal and policy implications of evidence-based practice

In many respects this chapter is the logical conclusion to the book, although this might not be immediately obvious. Our focus has been on the need for health professionals to base practice on current available evidence and, where there is no evidence, to generate some through research. This approach is predicated on the assumption that much of what is done in the provision of health care is not based on evidence. This admission is not helpful, of course, when health professionals endeavour to defend the care delivered to a patient or client. It is important to consider some policy and legal implications of evidence-based practice.

Trends

There are significant policy implications flowing from the emergence of evidence-based practice as a movement – and policy will always be informed by legal considerations. The likely trends in practice and health care delivery are being set in place right now. The emergence of evidence-based practice and the development of an evidence base for nursing, the pressure to introduce mechanisms for continuous quality improvement and its associated emphasis on outcome measures, together with the development of practice review techniques, are not accidents of fate. They all reflect a desire to deliver the best nursing care possible. Of course, there are some other goals such as cost containment, but those other aspirations tend to be the concern of managers rather than clinicians – even though we all have a vested interest in maximising the value for money element.

All innovations have the potential to bring with them unforeseen consequences and complications. Consider the following issues. As the evidence base for nursing is developed, questions arise about the nature of our obligation to utilise that evidence. Do we, for example, have a choice as to whether we apply the information in clinical guidelines and practice guidelines? Where we can identify gaps in the evidence, what is the nature of the obligation to fill the gaps? As national and international data sets become the norm, how will a failure to achieve a benchmark be construed at law? We need to think about these and many related issues.

At its root, the issue here is one of quality. It is reasonable to assume that the ambition of health professionals is to achieve the best possible outcome for those who come into our care. Thus, in an environment of practice based on evidence, it is the outcome of that practice with which we need to be concerned. In this chapter we have considered the various components of evidence-based practice. We have looked at the basic premise that there are deficiencies of available evidence and a failure to translate evidence into practice. We have looked at the assessment of that evidence, the application of that evidence and the ways in which the outcomes of that application can be evaluated.

Legal matters

The legal implications associated with the evidence-based approach are in no way an argument against it. However, launching the evidence-based practice movement has been rather like letting a genie out of a bottle: now it's out, it's never going back in! Having declared that our practice is largely not grounded on any evidence, we immediately highlight the obligation to generate evidence. This point will not be lost on the courts and legal profession.

The law takes a keen interest in the standard of care provided to consumers of health care services. It is instructive to consider just what the courts have actually said over the years on this subject. As one would expect, these comments have almost invariably been made in the context of negligence actions. The fact that the law has been established as a result of legal actions overwhelmingly involving doctors should provide little comfort at this point in time. Nurses are gaining increasing levels of autonomy in their practice in the pursuit of professionalisation. This means increasing levels of accountability, and in law accountability often translates into liability. Therefore, nurses – especially those who aspire to advanced and/or independent practice – cannot afford to be complacent about the possibility of litigation. This possibility has almost become probability, given the health care complaints mechanisms that are now in place in Australia and in many other countries. These comments pertain as much to allied health professionals as they do to nurses and medical practitioners, and recent experience has shown that they relate to all those who participate in the delivery of health services and at every level.

Negligence consists of conduct that is in breach of a legal duty of care because it falls below an accepted standard and results in harm. It is this 'accepted standard' with which we are concerned. We should be clear that not every slip or mistake amounts to negligence. The law does recognise – however unevenly – that accidents happen, and sometimes these accidents have unfortunate consequences. What the law requires is that reasonable care be provided in the circumstances. As practitioners, nurses need to know what constitutes reasonable care in the prevailing circumstances. This standard is expressed as the standard of care to which a reasonably careful, skilled and informed health professional would conform, even if that health professional is inexperienced.

In the case of *Bolam* v. *Friern Hospital Management Committee* [1957] 1 WLR 582, Mr Justice McNair stated (at p.57):

> *'A doctor is not guilty of negligence if he has acted in accordance with a practice accepted as proper by a responsible body of medical men skilled in that particular art ... Putting it the other way round, a man is not negligent, if he is acting in accordance with such a practice, merely because there is a body of opinion who would take a contrary view.'*

The effect of this judgment was that, for many years, the professions themselves determined standards. But even in Bolam's case, there was a caveat: the Court reserved the right to disapprove of any such professional standard if it believed it to be essentially misdirected. Of course, a defendant in such cases is judged on all the circumstances.

More recently, the influence in Australia of what has become known as the 'Bolam test' has waned. Cases such as *Albrighton* v. *Royal Prince Alfred Hospital* (1980) 2 NSWLR 542 and *F* v. *R* (1983) 33 SASR have diluted its force. In Albrighton's case, it was declared that the Bolam rule was:

> *'based on a wrong assumption that a jury should be directed that, if what is charged as negligence can be shown to have been done in accordance with the usual and customary practice and procedure ... they cannot find negligence. This ... is plainly wrong.'*

In the South Australian case of *F* v. *R*, the Chief Justice said:

> *'The Court has an obligation to scrutinise professional practices to ensure that they accord with the standard of reasonableness imposed by the law ... The ultimate question, however, is not whether the defendant's conduct accords with the practices of his profession or some part of it, but whether it conforms to the standard of reasonable care demanded by the law.'*

The Bolam test has also been challenged in other jurisdictions. Some American, Canadian and South African courts are dispensing with 'expert witnesses' in assessing the risk associated with a treatment or intervention and are instead using experts in appraising and interpreting research evidence. The Bolam test may no longer be good enough in a court of law, as the culture of evidence-based practice makes an impact. Scientific evidence presented in court will need to be more explicit and robust.

> **In practice . . .**
>
> Consider whether all practice other than that decreed to be best practice should be regarded as sub-standard practice and therefore, as negligent practice? What issue would this cast up for health care professionals? In the case of your friend the teacher, what would this mean?

The role of clinical practice guidelines

In determining whether a defendant health professional's conduct has fallen below that which is acceptable, it might well be relevant to consider industry standards or professional standards of practice. Such codes or standards have a great deal of evidentiary weight in ascertaining whether a breach of duty has occurred. So what about practice guidelines aimed at best practice?

In light of the position that courts have adopted to date, will practice guidelines or clinical guidelines be ignored by the courts in cases of alleged negligence? There is now some evidence to suggest the contrary. In fact, such guidelines might well become an alternative source of expert evidence. They might come to be regarded as a clear articulation of the benchmarks for appropriate care in a given situation.

Implications of evidence-based practice

The health care context has changed. Resources are becoming ever more scarce and economic rationalism – for no obvious reason – prevails as the dominant ethos. Privatisation, competition, the language of business and management: these are the contemporary tenets of health care services. Taking into account the views espoused by the courts to date, what might we expect as a consequence of evidence-based practice? Well, if the evidence is available, we had better apply it in our practice. If there is no evidence, we had better first establish why we are doing things the way we are, then seek to assemble evidence through research on care delivery outcomes.

There is no turning back. Notwithstanding the degree of contention surrounding evidence-based practice, it will have significant implications for the treatment of health care professionals who find themselves before the courts or complaints bodies. There are related policy implications for health care organisations at every level. In the same way as choosing not to use clinical and practice guidelines may not be an option for individual health professionals, choosing not to put in place policies and strategies may not be an option for organisations. To do so may constitute a breach of the non-delegable duty of care owed by health services to their clientele.

Health care takes the lead . . . and others follow

Evidence-based policy and practice is not confined to the world of health care. However, the dynamic and innovative principles and practices now being developed and utilised within the health care setting are breaking new ground and professionals from other disciplines are taking note.

Over the course of the twentieth century an increasingly educated, informed and questioning public has seen the demise of the unchallenged expert, regardless of profession. The nature of professional practice has therefore been required to evolve in order to ensure that practice is based on the evidence.

The determination of what 'counts' as evidence and strategies for the identification, appraisal, analysis and implementation of that evidence are issues that may be noted across many professions. These include not only health care, but education, criminal justice and urban planning, to name just a few.

The clinical practice of health care practitioners has often been the focus of much public attention, thus forcing them to examine in explicit detail not only 'what' they are doing, but also 'why'. As this book has attempted to demonstrate, this close scrutiny has necessitated the development of rigorous methodologies for the identification, appraisal, analysis and implementation of research evidence, including those that go beyond effectiveness to encompass feasibility, appropriateness meaningfulness and cost.

The education sector has certainly been quick to recognise the potential of this movement and the strides that health care has made toward resolving some of these issues. Just as in health care, education professionals seek to influence policy and change practice. They are also interested in more than just effectiveness, taking into account evidence that arises from the analysis of qualitative research when attempting to raise educational standards and processes.

The analysis and utilisation of evidence is quite clearly not a new concept for the field of criminal justice. As mentioned at the beginning of this book, several similarities can be identified between the processes of criminal justice and those of health care with regard to the identification and utilisation of evidence. The criminal justice system is similarly faced with issues regarding the review of available research evidence on topics such as effective strategies for the protection of the public and wider community, or the effective rehabilitation of repeat criminal offenders. As with health care, or any other discipline, criminal justice utilises a wide variety of research methods to inform practice. These methods need to be equally rigorous in order to establish the effectiveness of interventions. Similarly, the criminal justice system faces challenges with regard to implementation of guidelines derived from such research.

The complex nature of urban planning and policy (both politically and contextually) makes the idea of evidence-based practice far from straight forward. A wealth of research knowledge is available to urban planners and policy makers. Even so, however, there is significant debate regarding the potential of processes for the appraisal and synthesis of this information.

Davies et al. (2000) review some of the issues germane to research implementation across sectors and conclude that evidence of what works frequently has a disappointing impact on policy and practice across the public sector. They highlight the need, not only for the conduct of research initiatives, but also for strategies for effective implementation.

Professionals from any discipline do not function in isolation. Rapid and radical change in organisational structure has contributed to changing attitudes towards evidence-based practice. Communication and knowledge-sharing strategies are vital to the success of this movement. The sharing of insights and advances across sectors will generate different approaches as new challenges arise.

Consumer participation

Historically, it would seem that the agendas, priorities, interpretations and values of consumers have been at odds with those of the health profession, regardless of discipline. It appears, however, that this tide is turning. The future promises a collaborative approach to the process of evidence generation, review and utilisation in decision-making. 'Consumer participation' is the newest phase of the evidence-based movement as recent years have seen a shift both in consumer interest in this movement and in the interest of health professionals in the consumer perspective. While processes for encouraging consumer participation are still in their infancy, organisations that conduct systematic reviews of evidence and develop strategies for implementation are exploring ways of involving consumers in all aspects of these activities.

The facilitation of consumer participation in the evidence-based movement is complex and the challenges many. The risk of appearing tokenistic is ever present so it is important that genuine involvement is sought and legitimate partnerships are fostered. This will take time and genuine commitment from all key stakeholders. Although this 'real' participation may challenge traditional approaches to evidence generation, review and utilisation, it is desirable, logical and inevitable that consumer involvement holds a firm place in the future of evidence-based practice.

The National Health Service (NHS) in the United Kingdom proposes several elements that support a culture of consumer participation. These include an increased understanding and acceptance of the need to involve consumers, and ensuring that participants are assessed to determine whether or not they possess the requisite skills and resources to undertake consumer-based work. The NHS elements also include encouraging the development of a 'culture of partnership' in consumer involvement by seeking the cooperation of affiliated organisations and the voluntary sector to share in common endeavours; provision of appropriate training and support for professionals wanting to undertake patient involvement work along with support for consumers wishing to participate.

Finally, it is important to engender a commitment to consumer participation so that it is as highly regarded as any other activity of the organisation.

In short, the direction has been set and it is time for health professionals to take up the challenge of ensuring that consumers involved in this process are provided with the necessary tools and mechanisms of support to make a meaningful contribution.

In practice . . .

Does evidence-based health care represent the demise of the health professional, with prescriptive guidelines, clinical audits and an ever-increasing regulatory framework?

The rise and rise of information technology

The world is gradually being perceived as a single community united by means of rapid and comprehensive information systems. Modern communication and communication technologies have changed relationships between time and space, thus contributing to globalisation. New technologies, which enable rapid communication to take place in a number of different ways across the globe and permit information to be provided, sought and received on a scale hitherto unimaginable, have brought fundamental change to our lives.

Health care organisations are part of that global community and they are composed of highly distributed and complex structures and processes. As such, there is an increasingly large number of information interfaces between various health professionals, making efficient organisation of patient care and disease management significantly more complex. Innovative information technologies, such as clinical information systems, have the potential to support patient care by improving information logistics and information management.

Health professionals, administrators, policy makers and consumers all require information within the health care framework. Information technology is increasingly utilised in all health care domains and examples of this include patient administration systems and personnel, financial and wage systems. However, information technology in the health care environment is not restricted to management. Functional information requirements are also increasingly reliant on some form of information technology for their dissemination and utilisation in the clinical environment.

Clinical packages are utilised in a variety of health care settings, including pharmacy systems to monitor drug stocks, intensive care unit systems where patient data is captured from equipment or input by staff, and expert systems where a computer program assists the user to reach a diagnosis using rules derived originally from experts and increasingly from the best available evidence.

Issues surrounding the variation in units of care can be overcome by the successful implementation and utilisation of evidence-based information systems. The evidence-based health care movement endeavours to teach direct care professionals to evaluate research evidence and apply it to their clinical activities. It requires that the results of primary research be compiled in a methodical way and be made accessible to those involved in the decision-making process. It enhances knowledge by building on clinical expertise and verifiable facts regarding disease mechanisms.

Ultimately, evidence-based practice attempts to formalise the processes and principles that the best clinicians have perfected over time. Failure to utilise evidence systematically results in a considerable time lag before feasible, appropriate, meaningful and effective therapies come into use and others are withdrawn. Information systems that support evidence-based practice by capturing, transforming and maintaining data and knowledge are essential for efficient knowledge representation and information flow.

Health care is an information-intensive activity, and information technology, with its ability to store and retrieve information, can assist health professionals to synthesise the ever-increasing amounts of patient data and medical knowledge. In the health care environment, clinical information system requirements are growing as a result of risk management issues, standards of practice and external regulatory agency requirements.

Comprehensive information technology systems have the potential to provide health professionals with an alternative to time-consuming and ineffective manual documentation and data searching and collection methods. Information technology has the potential to change the nature of the work of health professionals, but it also presents implementation challenges because health professionals have been inadequately prepared to embrace this type of new technology and organisations have been inadequately prepared with a comprehensive implementation and evaluation process.

To a certain extent these issues are being overcome with software developments that not only provide access to evidence-based interventions and information, but also software to measure the success of its implementation. It is essential that there is continuous quality assessment of clinical information systems in order to ensure the ability of health professionals and health units to see that their systems reach their full potential in an ever changing and evolving environment. Facilitation of review and trend analysis of direct and indirect inputs to patient care and differences in practice and patterns of care in different areas is of significance. This includes ensuring that the appropriate technology is utilised and updated as frequently as possible.

It is the implementation of innovations such as these that will contribute to more effective communication regarding health care interventions between health professionals, thus resulting in:

- Better patient outcomes
- Standardised practice resulting in a reduction in errors and improved compliance with guidelines
- Less variation in practice leading to less variation in patient outcomes and the cost of health care
- Continuous quality monitoring and improvement

In order for health care organizations to be successful in their endeavour to achieve evidence-based health care, they need to realise the necessity of linking their information systems to organisational improvement. Health care executives need to take advantage of the current wave of new and innovative clinical information systems. They need to make information system improvements through system analysis, developing a strategic vision, allocating necessary funds and monitoring the organisation's information system while exploring potential improvements.

Conclusion

Practice, policy and legal pressures are all impelling health professionals and indeed professionals from other sectors towards evidence-based practice. It is likely that evidence-based practice is here to stay, and probable that it will become the norm. It would be difficult to mount a persuasive case that it should be otherwise. In time, the evidence base will grow and the various disciplines will be richer as a result. The future of evidence-based practice will see the use of information that is cumulative and evolutionary, rather than information that is static.

Evidence-based information will play a central and vital role in decision-making for professionals and consumers in a diverse range of settings, both clinical and otherwise. The ways in which evidence is gathered, appraised and utilised has come a considerable way, and the journey continues.

The JBI Model of Evidence-Based Health Care has been constructed to enable reasoning and critique about evidence-based health care and its role in improving global health, within a logical conceptual framework. Drawn from the experience of the Joanna Briggs Institute and its global partners in promoting and facilitating evidence-based health care across the world, it is an attempt to conceptually represent the components of a cyclical process that is both responsive to priorities in global health and, in turn, serves to improve global health.

The model posits that evidence-based practice involves giving consideration to the best available evidence; the context in which the care is delivered; client preference; and the professional judgment of the health professional. Promoting and facilitating evidence-based health care is depicted as consisting of four major components of the evidence-based health care process:

- Health care evidence generation
- Evidence synthesis
- Evidence/knowledge transfer
- Evidence utilisation

Each of these components is modelled to incorporate three essential elements, and the achievement of improved global health is conceptualised as both the goal or endpoint of any or all of the model components and the *raison d'être* and driver of evidence-based health care. Central to the model is a pluralistic approach to what constitutes legitimate evidence; an inclusive approach to evidence appraisal, extraction and synthesis; the importance of effective and appropriate transfer of evidence; and the complexity of evidence utilisation.

The exploration of new and innovative approaches to evidence-based practice is ongoing and we hope that you share our enthusiasm for the development, provision and consumption of evidence-based care.

In practice . . .

So what does this really mean in practical terms for the health professional who goes to work in the clinical environment every day? You are required to make decisions regarding treatment and care of other individuals daily, and in order to make informed decisions you need to ensure that you have the best available evidence. Regardless of whether you are involved in these processes actively or passively, you have a contribution to make to evidence-based practice in your clinical environment. You may not be involved in the systematic review process or even in guideline development, but you will be required to utilise such information in your practice, so it is important that you have a comprehensive understanding of the theories and concepts behind that information. Hopefully this text has provided you with both the theory and its practical application thereby *making evidence meaningful* for you.

Further reading and resources

If you are interested in learning more about the trends and possibilities for the future addressed in this chapter, we would suggest the following:

Davies, H., Nutley, S. M., and Smith, P. C. (2001) *What Works? Evidence-Based Policy and Practice in Public Services*. Polity Press, Bristol, United Kingdom.

Forrester, K. and Griffiths, D. (2001) *Essentials of Law for Health Professionals*. Harcourt Publishers International, Sydney, Australia.

References

Allen, D. (1985) Nursing research and social control: alternative models of science that emphasise understanding and emancipation. *Journal of Nursing Scholarship* **17** (2): 58–64.

Allen, D., Benner, P. et al. (1986) Three paradigms for nursing research: methodological implications. In: Chin, P. (ed.) *Nursing Research Methodology*, pp. 23–38. Washington DC, Aspen Systems.

Audi, R. (1995) *The Cambridge Dictionary of Philosophy*. Cambridge, Cambridge University Press.

Avis, M. (1994) Reading research critically II. An introduction to appraisal: assessing the evidence. *Journal of Clinical Nursing* **3** (5): 271–7.

Bastian, H. (1996) Raising the standard: practice guidelines and consumer participation. *International Journal of Quality in Health Care* **8** (5): 485–90.

Bauman, Z. (1978) *Hermeneutics and Social Science: Approaches to Understanding*. London, Hutchinson.

Berger, P. and Luckman, T. (1971) *The Social Construction of Reality: A Treatise in the Sociology of Knowledge*. Harmondsworth, Penguin.

Bernstein, R. (1986) *The Restructuring of Social and Political Theory*. Oxford, Blackwell.

Botha, M. (1989) Theory development in perspective: the role of conceptual frameworks and models in theory development. *Journal of Advanced Nursing* **14** (1): 49–55.

Burnett, A. and Winyard, G. (1998) Clinical audit at the heart of clinical effectiveness. *Journal of Quality in Clinical Practice* **18** (1): 3–19.

Cannon, S. (1989) Social research in stressful settings: difficulties for the sociologist studying the treatment of breast cancer. *Sociology of Health and Illness* **11** (1): 66–77.

Carande-Kulis, V. G., Maciosek, M. V., Briss, P. A., Teutsch, S. M., Zaza, S., Truman, B. I. et al. (2000) Methods for systematic reviews of economic evaluations for the Guide to Community Preventive Services. Task Force on Community Preventive Services. *American Journal of Preventive Medicine* **18** (1 Suppl): 75–91.

Centre for Reviews and Dissemination (1999) Getting evidence into practice. *Effective Health Care Bulletin* 5: 1–16.

Chessick, R. (1980) The problematical self in Kant and Kohut. *Psychoanal. Q* (49): 456–73.

Chin, P. and Jacobs, M. (1987) *Theory in Nursing: A Systematic Approach*. St Louis, Mosby.

Cochrane, A. (1979) 1931–1971: a critical review, with particular reference to the medical profession. *Medicines for the Year 2000*, pp. 1–11. London, Office of Health Economics.

Davies, H., Nutley, S. et al. (2000) *What works? Evidence Based Policy and Practice in Public Services*. Bristol, Polity Press.

Davis, D., Evani, M., Jadad, A. et al. (2003) The case for knowledge translation: shortening the journey from evidence to effect. *British Medical Journal* 327: 33–5.

Dawes, M., Davies, P. et al. (1999) *Evidence Based Practice: A Primer for Health Care Professionals*. London, Churchill Livingstone.

Dawes, M., Summerskill, W., Glasziou, P., Cartabellotta, A., Martin, J., Hopayian, K. et al. (2005) Sicily statement on evidence-based practice. *BMC Medical Education* 5: 1.

Denzin, N. and Lincoln, Y. (1994) *Handbook of Qualitative Research*. Thousand Oaks, CA, Sage.

Dicenso, A. and Cullum, N. (1998) Implementing evidence-based nursing: some misconceptions. *Evidence-Based Nursing* **1** (2): 38–40.

Dickinson, V. (1998) Moving audit into midwifery practice. *Practising Midwife* **7** (8): 14–18.

Dixon-Woods, M. and Fitzpatrick, R. (2001) Qualitative research in systematic reviews has established a place for itself. *British Medical Journal* **323** (7316): 765–6.

Eccles, M., Mason, J. et al. (2000) Developing valid cost effectiveness guidelines: a methodological report from the North of England evidence based guideline development project. *Quality in Health Care* **9** (2): 127–32.

Emden, C. and Sandelowski, M. (1998) The good, the bad and the relative, part one: conceptions of goodness in qualitative research. *International Journal of Nursing Practice* **4** (4): 206–12.

Evans, D. and Pearson, A. (2001) Systematic reviews: gatekeepers of nursing knowledge. *Journal of Clinical Nursing* **10** (5): 593–9.

Fay, B. (1975) *Social Theory and Political Practice*. London, Allen & Unwin.

Garland, G. and Corfield, F. (1999) Audit. In: Hamer, S. and Collinson, G. (eds) *Achieving Evidence Based Practice: A Handbook for Practitioners*, pp. 129–151. London, Baillière Tindall.

GL '99 (1999) Fourth International Conference on Grey Literature, Washington, DC, October 1999 <www.nyam.org/library/greywhat.shtml> (accessed 31 March 2005).

Glaser, B. and Strauss, A. (1967) *The Discovery of Grounded Theory: Strategies for Qualitative Research*. Chicago, IL, Aldine.

Grimshaw, J., Shirran, L., Thomas, R., Mowatt, G., Fraser, C., Bero, L. et al. (2001) Changing provider behaviour: an overview of systematic reviews of interventions. *Medical Care* **39** (Supplement 2): 11.2–11.45.

Haddow, G., Watts, R. and Robertson, J. (2005) Effectiveness of a pelvic floor muscle exercise program on urinary incontinence following childbirth. *International Journal of Evidence Based Healthcare* **3** (5).

Hodgkinson, B., Evans, D. and O'Neill, S. (2000) *Knowledge Retention from Pre-operative Patient Information: A Systematic Review*. The Joanna Briggs Institute for Evidence-Based Nursing and Midwifery.

Humphris, D. (1999) Types of evidence. In: Hamer, S. and Collinson, G. (eds) *Achieving Evidence Based Practice: A Handbook for Practitioners*, pp. 13–39. London, Baillière Tindall.

Hutchinson, A. and Baker, R. (1999) *Making Use of Guidelines in Clinical Practice*. Abingdon, Oxon, Radcliffe Medical Press Ltd.

Johnson, M. and Griffiths, R. (2001) Developing evidence based clinicians. *International Journal of Nursing Practice* **7** (2): 109–18.

Jones, T. (2000) *Effectiveness of Mechanical Compression Devices in Attaining Hemostasis after Removal of a Femoral Sheath following Femoral Artery Cannulation for Cardiac Interventional Procedures: A Systematic Review*. The Joanna Briggs Institute for Evidence-Based Nursing and Midwifery.

Kelley, D. and Connor, D. (1979) The emotional cycle of change. In: Jones, J. and Pfieffer, J. (eds) *The Annual Handbook for Group Facilitators*, pp. 117–22. LaJolla, CA, University Associates.

Kenrick, M. and Luker, K. (1996) An exploration of the influence of managerial factors on research utilisation in district nursing practice. *Journal of Advanced Nursing* **23** (4): 697–704.

Kinn, S. (1995) Clinical audit: a tool for nursing practice. *Nursing Standard* **9** (15): 35–6.

Kitson, A., Harvey, G. et al. (1998) Enabling the implementation of evidence based practice: a conceptual framework. *Quality in Health Care* **7** (3): 149–58.

Light, D. and Pillemer, B. (1984) *Summing Up: The Science of Reviewing Research.* Harvard University Press, Cambridge, MA.

Lippitt, G. (1973) *Visualising Change: Model Building and the Change Process.* LaJolla, CA, University Associates.

MacPherson, K. (1983) Feminist methods: a new paradigm for nursing research. *Advances in Nursing Science* **5** (2): 17–25.

McHoul, A. and Grace, W. (1993) *A Foucault Primer: Discourse, Power and the Subject.* Melbourne, Melbourne University Press.

Mitchell, L. (1998) We must recognise change as a way of life. *Healthcare Finance Management* **52** (6): 48–50, 52, 54.

Moher, D., Jadad, A. et al. (1995) Assessing the quality of randomised controlled trials: an annotated bibliography of scales and checklists. *Controlled Clinical Trials* **16**: 62–73.

Morgan, L. and Fennessy, G. (1996) How to undertake clinical audit: a new service. *Nursing Standard* **10** (5): 32–3.

Morrell, C. and Harvey, G. (1999) *The Clinical Audit Handbook: Improving the Quality of Health Care.* London, Baillière Tindall.

Muir-Gray, J. (2001) *Evidence Based Health Care: How to Make Health Policy and Management Decisions.* London, Churchill Livingstone.

Munhall, P. and Oiler, C. (1986) *Nursing Research: A Qualitative Perspective.* Connecticut, Appleton Century Crofts.

Nagy, S., Lumby, J. et al. (2001) Nurses' beliefs about the conditions that hinder or support evidence based nursing. *International Journal of Nursing Practice* 7: 314–21.

National Centre for Clinical Audit (1997) *Key Points from Audit Literature Related to Criteria for Clinical Audit.* London, NCCA.

NHMRC (1999) *How to Present the Evidence for Consumers: Preparation of Consumer Publications.* Canberra, National Health and Medical Research Council.

NHMRC (2000) *How to Put the Evidence into Practice: Implementation and Dissemination Strategies.* Canberra, National Health and Medical Research Council.

NHS Executive (1998) A First Class Service: Quality in the New NHS. London: Department of Health.

Nicklin, W. and McVeety, J. (2002) Canadian nurses describe their perceptions of patient safety in teaching hospitals. Wake up call! *Canadian Journal of Nursing Leadership.*

Nixon, J., Duffy, S. et al. (2004) The usefulness of the NHS Economic Evaluation Databse to researchers undertaking technology assessment reviews. *International Journal of Technology Assessment in Health Care* **20** (3): 249–57.

Noblit, G. and Hare, R. (1998) *Meta-ethnography: Synthesising Qualitative Studies.* Newbury Park, Sage.

Nutbeam, D. and Harris, E. (1999) *Theory in a Nutshell: A Guide to Health Promotion Theory.* Sydney, McGraw Hill Australia.

Oakley, A. (1981) *Interviewing Women: A Contradiction in Terms.* In: Roberts, H. (ed.) *Doing Feminist Research.* London, Routledge.

Pathman, D. E., Konrad, T. R., Freed, G. L., Freeman, V. A. and Koch, G. G. (1996) The awareness-to-adherence model of the steps to clinical guideline compliance: the case of paediatric vaccine recommendations. *Medical Care* 34: 873–89.

Pearsall, J. and Trumble, B. (eds) (1995) *The Oxford Encyclopedic Dictionary*, 2nd edn. New York, Oxford University Press.

Pearson, A. (1998) Excellence in care: future dimensions for effective nursing. *Nursing Times* 3: 25–7.

Pearson, A. (1999) Evidence based nursing: quality through research. In: Nay, R. and Garrett, S. (eds) *Nursing Older People: Issues and Innovations,* pp. 338–52. Sydney, McLennan and Petty.

Pearson, A. (2002) Nursing takes the lead: re-defining what counts as evidence in Australian health care. *Reflections on Nursing Leadership Fourth Quarter* 37: 18–21.

Pearson, A. (2003) Liberating our conceptualisation of 'evidence'. *Journal of Advanced Nursing* 44: 441–2.

Pearson, A. (2004) Balancing the evidence: incorporating the synthesis of qualitative data into systematic reviews. *JBI Reports* 2: 45–64.

Pearson, A., Wiechula, R., Lockwood, C. and Court, A. (2005) The JBI Model of Evidence-Based Health Care. *International Journal of Evidence Based Health Care* 3: 207–15.

Pignone, M., Saha, S., Hoerger, T., Lohr, K. N., Teutsch, S. and Mandelblatt, J. (2005) Challenges in systematic reviews of economic analyses. *Annals of Internal Medicine* **142** (12): 1073–9.

Popay, J., Rogers, A. et al. (1998) Rationale and standards for the systematic review of qualitative literature in health services research. *Qualitative Health Research* **8** (3): 341–51.

Rogers, E. (1983) *Diffusion of Innovations*. New York, Free Press.

Sackett, D., Richardson, W. et al. (1997) *Evidence Based Medicine: How to Practice and Teach Evidence Based Medicine*. New York, Churchill Livingstone.

Sackett, D. and Rosenberg, W. (1995) The need for evidence based medicine. *Journal of the Royal Society of Medicine* **88** (11): 620–4.

Sackett, D., Rosenberg, W., Gray, J. A., Haynes, R. B. and Richardson, W. S. (1996) Evidence based medicine: what it is and what it isn't. *British Medical Journal* **312** (7023): 71–2.

Sanson-Fisher, R. W. (2004) Diffusion of innovation theory for clinical change. *Medical Journal of Australia* **180** (6 Suppl.): S55–S56.

Schwartz, H. and Jacobs, J. (1979) *Qualitative Sociology: A Method to the Madness*. New York, Free Press.

Soumerai, S., McLaughlin, T. et al. (1998) Effect of local medical opinion leaders on quality of care for acute myocardial infarction: a randomized controlled trial. *Journal of the American Medical Association* **279** (17): 1392–4.

Stanley, L. and Wise, S. (1983) *Breaking Out: Feminist Consciousness and Feminist Research*. London, Routledge & Kegan Paul.

Starr, J. (1982) Towards a social phenomenology of aging: studying the self process in biographical work. *International Journal of Aging and Human Development* **16** (4): 255–70.

Stern, C. and Lockwood, C. (2005) Knowledge retention from pre-operative patient information. *International Journal of Evidence Based Healthcare* 3 (3).

Taylor, S. J. and Bogdan, R. (1984). *Introduction to Qualitative Research Methods: The Search for Meaning* (2nd edn). New York, John Wiley & Sons.

Taylor, S. J. and Bogdan, R. (1998) *Introduction to Qualitative Research Methods: A Guidebook and Resource* (3rd edn). New York, Wiley.

Thompson, C. and Thompson, G. (1998) Supporting carers of people with Alzheimer's type dementia – a review of the evidence of effectiveness. Cochrane Database of Systematic Reviews. Cochrane Library Issue 2.

Thompson, C. et al. (2001) The accessibility of research-based knowledge for nurses in United Kingdom acute care settings. *Journal of Advanced Nursing* **36** (1): 11–22.

Trinder, L. and Reynolds, S. (2000) *Evidence Based Practice: A Critical Appraisal*. Oxford, Blackwell Science Ltd.

Winstead-Fry, P. (1980) The scientific method and its impact on holistic health. *Advances in Nursing Science* **2**: 1–7.

Further Reading

Burnett, J., Grimmer, K. et al. (2005) Development of a generic critical appraisal tool by consensus: presentation of first round Delphi survey results. *International Journal of Allied Health Sciences and Practice* **3** (1).

Centre for Reviews and Dissemination (2001) Undertaking Systematic Reviews of Effectiveness. *CRD Report Number 4* (2nd edn). NHS Centre for Reviews and Dissemination, York.

Dobrow, M. J., Goel, V. and Upshur, R. E. G. (2004) Evidence-based health policy: context and utilisation. *Science & Medicine* **58** (1): 207–17.

Fernandez, R., Griffiths, R. and Murie, P. (2003) Comparison of late night and early morning removal of short term urethral catheters – a systematic review. *JBI Reports* 1: 1–16.

Forrester, K. and Griffiths, D. (2001) *Essentials of Law for Health Professionals.* New South Wales, Harcourt Publishers International.

Habermas, J. (1971) *Knowledge and Human Interests.* Boston, MA, Beacon Press.

Joanna Briggs Institute (2001) Maintaining oral hydration in older people. Evidence Based Practice Information Sheets for Health Professionals, Volume 5, Issue 1.

Johnston, G., Crombie, I. et al. (2000) Reviewing audit: barriers and facilitating factors in closing the audit loop. *Quality in Health Care* 9: 23–36.

Miller, S. and Fredericks, M. (2003) The nature of evidence in qualitative research methods. *International Journal of Qualitative Methods* **2** (1) Article 4 (www.ualberta.ca/~ijqm) (accessed 1 September 2005).

NHMRC (1999) *A Guide to the Development, Implementation and Evaluation of Clinical Practice Guidelines.* Canberra, National Health and Medical Research Council.

Stetler, C. B. (1983) Nurses and research responsibility and involvement. *National Intravenous Therapy Associations, Inc.* **6** (May/June): 207–12.

Stetler, C. B. (1985) Research utilization: defining the concept. *Image: The Journal of Nursing Scholarship* **17** (2): 40–4.

Stetler, C. B. (1994) Refinement of the Stelter/Marram model for application of research findings to practice. *Nursing Outlook*, January/February, 15–25.

Stetler, C. B. and Marram, G. (1976) Evaluating research findings for applicability in practice. *Nursing Outlook* **24** (9), 559–63.

Stevens, K. R. (2002) ACE Star Model of EBP. *The Cycle of Knowledge Transformation.* Academic Center for Evidence-based Practice (www.acestar.uthscsa.edu).

Thompson, C. and Spilsbury, K. (2004) Support for carers of people with Alzheimer's type dementia. *Cochrane Database of Systematic Reviews* 4.

Thorne, S., Jensen, L., Kearney, M. H., Noblit, G. and Sandelowski, M. (2004) Qualitative metasynthesis: reflections on methodological orientation and ideological agenda. *Qualitative Health Research* **14** (10): 1342–65.

Titler, M. G. and Everett, L. Q. (2001) Translating research into practice: considerations for critical care investigators. *Critical Care Nursing Clinics of North America* **13** (4): 587–604.

West, B., Wimpenny, P., Duff, L., Macduff, C., Lyon, M. and Rae, K. (2001) An educational initiative to promote the use of clinical guidelines in nursing practice. *National Board for Nursing Midwifery and Health Visiting* (Scotland), Edinburgh.

Winter, R. and Munn-Giddings, C. (2001) *A Handbook for Action Research in Health and Social Care.* Routledge, London.

Appendix 1

Systematic Review Protocol Example: Smoking Cessation Interventions and Strategies for Hospitalised Patients

J. Briggs

Background

Smoking has been identified as the primary cause of avoidable death and disease when compared with all other drugs used in Australia (NHMRC, 1991). Evidence on the potential risks of smoking was first identified nearly 60 years ago. In 1991 the Federal Court determined that passive exposure to cigarette smoke could cause lung cancer, asthma and respiratory disease. There has also been a significant increase in public support for measures designed to reduce the exposure to tobacco smoke. Despite the increase in public knowledge, and the momentum gained for smoke-exposure reduction, the prevalence of smoking continues to represent a threat to the health and well-being of active and passive smokers alike. Programmes that encourage smokers to quit have been described as the most significant factors in promoting health and reducing the burden of disease related to smoking in Australia. Smoking cessation has a measurable impact on health improvement. Within two to three years of quitting, ex-smokers are at a significantly lower risk of myocardial infarction or stroke.

Despite the significance of the impact of cessation programmes on smoking, many smokers enter and exit the health care system every day without receiving advice about this important health risk. Smoking cessation interventions offer clinicians and health care providers a significant opportunity to improve current and future health-related outcomes. It is essential, therefore, that health care providers, including clinicians, smoking cessation specialists, health care administrators and health care purchasers take an active role in reducing the prevalence of tobacco use. One way to do this is through the support and delivery of effective smoking cessation interventions (Fiore et al., 1996). It is timely and essential, therefore, to provide clinicians with the best available evidence on currently available interventions for hospitalised smokers. There is now clear evidence for the effectiveness of a number of smoking cessation interventions readily available to health care workers, particularly primary health care professionals. There is also good evidence that the use of guidelines for smoking cessation can significantly increase quit rates (Grimshaw et al., 1995; Worrall et al., 1997).

Review questions

This review seeks to establish, through the available literature, what is best practice for smoking cessation. The specific review questions to be addressed are:

(1) What constitutes current best practice in relation to smoking cessation interventions for hospitalised patients?
(2) What are the indications for, and the safety and effectiveness of, the range of interventions available for hospitalised patients?

Inclusion criteria

Types of participants

This review will consider all studies that involve human subjects of any age who smoke. Although the review is to be focused on hospitalised patients who smoke, studies using non-hospitalised participants will also be considered where the interventions could be applied in the hospital setting.

Types of intervention

Interventions of interest included those related to the efficacy and/or effectiveness of smoking cessation programmes including screening systems; assessment strategies; intervention programmes; specific clinical interventions; and follow-up assessment strategies.

Types of outcome measure

The primary outcome of interest is smoking cessation. Secondary outcomes include smoking reduction, withdrawal symptoms, weight gain, and intervention-specific side effects.

Types of studies

The review considered all studies evaluating the effectiveness or efficacy of interventions/strategies relating to smoking cessation in the hospitalised patient. In the absence of this type of study, those that evaluate interventions and programmes that may readily be applied to the hospitalised patient will also be considered.

Search strategy

The search strategy will be designed to access both published and unpublished materials and will comprise three stages:

(1) A limited search of CINAHL and Medline to identify relevant keywords contained in the title, abstract and subject descriptors.
(2) Terms identified in this way, and the synonyms used by respective databases, will be used in an extensive search of the literature.
(3) Reference lists and bibliographies of the articles collected from those identified in stage two above will be searched.

The initial search terms will be 'smoking', 'cessation', 'reduction' and 'withdrawal'. Articles published in the last 10 years in English and indexed in the following databases will be searched:

CINAHL	Embase
Medline	Cancerlit
Current Contents	DARE
Cochrane Library	Web search – metacrawler
PsycINFO	

Full copies of articles identified by the search, and considered to meet the inclusion criteria, based on their title, abstract and subject descriptors, will be obtained for data synthesis. Articles identified through reference list and bibliographic searches will also be considered for data collection based on their title. Two reviewers will independently select articles against the inclusion criteria. Discrepancies in reviewer selections will be resolved at a meeting between reviewers prior to selected articles being retrieved.

Critical appraisal

Identified studies that meet the publication criteria will be grouped into one of the following categories: experimental studies, cohort studies, case control studies, interpretive and critical studies, cost minimisation studies and textual/opinion papers. These studies will then be assessed independently for methodological validity by two reviewers, prior to inclusion in the review using the corresponding checklist from the SUMARI suite developed by the Joanna Briggs Institute (Appendix 2). Any disagreements that arise between the reviewers will be resolved through discussion and with the assistance of a third reviewer where required.

Data collection

Following assessment of methodological quality, the papers will be grouped according to whether they are quantitative, qualitative or opinion-based. A data extraction tool has been developed specifically for quantitative research data extraction based on the work of the Cochrane Collaboration and the Centre for Reviews and Dissemination (Appendix 3). Qualitative research data and expert opinion will be extracted using the data extraction tools developed for the

SUMARI software suite (Appendix 3). Two reviewers will independently perform data extraction.

Data synthesis

For quantitative data, where possible, odds ratio (for categorical outcome data) or standardised mean differences (for continuous data) and their 95% confidence intervals will be calculated from the data generated by each included randomised controlled trial. If appropriate with available data, results from comparable groups of studies will be pooled into statistical meta-analysis using Review Manager software from the Cochrane Collaboration. Heterogeneity between combined studies will be tested using standard chi-square test. Where statistical pooling is not possible the findings will be presented in narrative form.

For qualitative data, where meta-synthesis is possible, textual data will be pooled using the Qualitative Assessment and Review Instrument (JBI-QARI) and Narrative, Opinion and Text Assessment and Review Instrument (JBI-NOTARI) package from the SUMARI software suite. Where textual pooling is not possible the findings will be presented in narrative form.

References

NHMRC (1991) *National Health Policy on Tobacco in Australia and Examples of Strategies for Implementation*, National Health and Medical Research Council, Canberra.

Fiore, M. C., Bailey, W. C., Cohen, S. J. et al. *Smoking cessation: Clinical Practice Guideline No 18*. Rockville, MD: US Department of Health and Human Services, Public Health Service. Agency for Health Care Policy and Research. AHCPR Publication No. 96-0692. April 1996.

Grimshaw, J., Freemantle, N. et al. (1995). Developing and implementing clinical practice guidelines. *Quality Health Care* 4: 55–64.

Worrall, G., Chaulk, P., et al. (1997) The effects of clinical practice guidelines on patient outcomes in primary care: a systematic review [see comments]. *Canadian Medical Association Journal* **156** (12): 1705–12.

Appendix 2
Critical Appraisal Tools

JBI Critical Appraisal Checklist for Experimental Studies

Reviewer _____ Date _____

Author _____ Year _____ Record number _____

	Yes	No	Unclear
1. Was the assignment to treatment groups random?			
2. Were participants blinded to treatment allocation?			
3. Was allocation to treatment groups concealed from the allocator?			
4. Were the outcomes of people who withdrew described and included in the analysis?			
5. Were those assessing outcomes blind to the treatment allocation?			
6. Were the control and treatment groups comparable at entry?			
7. Were groups treated identically other than for the named interventions?			
8. Were outcomes measured in the same way for all groups?			
9. Were outcomes measured in a reliable way?			
10. Was there adequate follow-up (>80%)?			
11. Was appropriate statistical analysis used?			

Overall appraisal: Include ☐   Exclude ☐   Seek further info. ☐

Comments (Including reasons for exclusion)

_____

_____

_____

JBI QARI Critical Appraisal Checklist for Interpretive and Critical Research

Reviewer _____   Date _____
Author _____ Year _____   Record number _____

	Yes	**No**	**Unclear**
1. Is there congruity between the stated philosophical perspective and the research methodology?			
2. Is there congruity between the research methodology and the research question or objectives?			
3. Is there congruity between the research methodology and the methods used to collect data?			
4. Is there congruity between the research methodology and the representation and analysis of data?			
5. Is there congruity between the research methodology and the interpretation of results?			
6. Is there a statement locating the researcher culturally or theoretically?			
7. Is the influence of the researcher on the research, and vice-versa, addressed?			
8. Are participants, and their voices, adequately represented?			
9. Is the research ethical according to current criteria or, for recent studies, is there evidence of ethical approval by an appropriate body?			
10. Do the conclusions drawn in the research report flow from the analysis, or interpretation, of the data?			

Overall appraisal: Include ☐   Exclude ☐   Seek further info. ☐

Comments (including reasons for exclusion)

_____
_____
_____

JBI NOTARI Critical Appraisal Checklist for Narrative, Opinion and Textual Papers

Reviewer _____   Date _____

Author _____   Year _____   Record number _____

	Yes	**No**	**Unclear**
1. Is the source of the opinion clearly identified?			
2. Does the source of the opinion have standing in the field of expertise?			
3. Are the interests of patients the central focus of the opinion?			
4. Is the opinion's basis in logic/experience clearly argued?			
5. Is there reference to the extant literature/evidence and any incongruence with it logically defended?			
6. Is the opinion supported by peers?			

Overall appraisal: Include ☐   Exclude ☐   Seek further info. ☐

Comments (including reasons for exclusion)

_____

_____

_____

JBI Critical Appraisal Checklist for Observational Studies

Reviewer _____   Date _____

Author _____   Year _____   Record number _____

	Yes	No	Unclear	N/A
1. Is the study based on a random or pseudo-random sample?				
2. Are the criteria for inclusion in the sample clearly defined?				
3. Were outcomes assessed using objective criteria?				
4. If comparisons are being made, was there sufficient description of the groups?				
5. Was an appropriate statistical analysis used?				

Overall appraisal: Include ☐   Exclude ☐   Seek further info. ☐

Comments (including reasons for exclusion)

_____

_____

_____

Checklist for Assessing the Validity of Cohort Studies

Reviewer _____   Date _____

Author _____   Year _____   Record number _____

	Yes	**No**	**Unclear**
1. Is sample representative of patients in the population as a whole?			
2. Are the patients at a similar point in the course of their condition/illness?			
3. Are outcomes assessed using objective criteria?			
4. Was follow-up carried out over a sufficient time period?			
5. Were the outcomes of people who withdrew described and included in the analysis?			
6. Were outcomes measured in a reliable way?			
7. Was appropriate statistical analysis used?			

Overall appraisal: Include ☐   Exclude ☐   Seek further info. ☐

Comments (including reasons for exclusion)

_____

_____

_____

Checklist for Assessing the Validity of Case Control Studies

Reviewer _____   Date _____

Author _____   Year _____   Record number _____

	Yes	**No**	**Unclear**
1. Are confounding factors identified and strategies to deal with them stated?			
2. Has bias been minimised in relation to selection of cases and of controls?			
3. Were outcomes assessed using objective criteria?			
4. Were the outcomes of people who withdrew described and included in the analysis?			
5. Were outcomes measured in a reliable way?			
6. Was appropriate statistical analysis used?			

Overall appraisal: Include ☐   Exclude ☐   Seek further info. ☐

Comments (including reasons for exclusion)

_____

_____

_____

Appendix 3

Data Extraction Tools

JBI Data Extraction Form for Experimental/Observational Studies

Reviewer _____   Date _____

Author _____   Year _____

Journal _____   Record number _____

Study method   RCT   Quasi-RCT   Longitudinal

Retrospective   Observational   Other _____

Participants

Setting   _____

Population   _____

Sample size

Intervention 1 _____   Intervention 2 _____   Intervention 3 _____

Interventions

Intervention 1 _____

_____

Intervention 2 _____

_____

Intervention 3 _____

_____

Clinical outcome measures

Outcome description	Scale/measure

Study results

(a) Dichotomous data

Outcome	Intervention ( ) number/total number	Intervention ( ) number/total number

(b) Continuous data

Outcome	Intervention ( ) mean & SD (number)	Intervention ( ) mean & SD (number)

Authors' conclusions

_____

_____

Comments

_____

_____

JBI QARI Data Extraction Form for Interpretive and Critical Research

Reviewer _____   Date _____

Author   _____   Year _____

Journal _____   Record number _____

Study description

Methodology _____

Method _____

Intervention _____

Setting _____

Geographical _____

Cultural _____

Participants _____

Data analysis _____

Authors' conclusions

_____

_____

Comments

_____

_____

Findings	Illustration from publication (page number)	Evidence		
		Unequivocal	Credible	Unsupported

Extraction of findings complete YES/NO

JBI NOTARI Data Extraction Form

Reviewer _____   Date _____

Author _____   Year _____

Journal _____   Record number _____

Study description

Type of text _____

Stated _____

Allegiance/position _____

Intervention _____

Setting _____

Geographical _____

Cultural _____

Logic of argument _____

Data analysis _____

Authors' conclusions

_____

Comments

_____

Findings	Illustration from Publication (page number)	Evidence		
		Unequivocal	Credible	Unsupported

Extraction of findings complete YES/NO

Index

action plan 146–7
action research 47–8, 131
action theory 42
aetiology 63
Agency for Healthcare Quality Research
 (AHQR) 103, 115–16, 152
allied health professions 10, 104, 124–5
 appendices 102
 appraisal, critical criteria 77–8
 economic evaluation studies 83–6
 expert opinion 86–8
 guidelines 113–14
 purpose, meaningfulness 89
 randomised controlled trials (RCTs) 76,
  77–8
 systematic reviews 74–5
 validity criteria 80, 81, 83
 see also tools
Appraisal of Guidelines Research and
 Evaluation (AGREE) 113
appropriateness
 defined 20, 28, 29, 64
 evidence sources 49
 interventions 92
 model 18, 20, 36, 96–7, 111, 154
 recommendations 102
 sources 86–7
 study method 78–9
 see also validity
Aristotle 47
article retrieval 70
 see also database searching
assessment
 clinical question source 63
 criteria 61–2, 80
 database 66
 research quality 61–2
 standards 81
 system 96–7, 175, 176
 tool, effectiveness 151
 validity 86
audit, clinical
 cycle 142
 feedback process 129, 130, 138,
  147
 goals 140
 key stages 141–8

methodology 149
planning 141–2, 146
process, described 141
re-auditing 147
report writing 148–9
research links 151
strategies 148
tools 149–51
Audit-maker 150
Australasian Cochrane Centre 7
Australian Centre for Evidence-based
 Clinical Practice 150
Austrom database 66

balance 30–1, 40
barriers to change 104, 115, 119, 120–2
behaviour changing 129, 147
best available evidence 6, 8, 32, 64, 86
bias 48–9, 75–7, 80, 81
blinding 75, 76, 78
Bolam test 160–2
Boolean operators 67
budget preparation 135

care standards
 best practice 6, 9, 142–3, 144
 dissemination 107, 144
 establishment 140
 legal matters 156, 158, 159–60
 negligence 160–2
 quality 113, 139, 159
 see also guidelines
case control studies 79–80, 182
category defined 96
CDSS (clinical decision support system)
 128
Centre for Evidence-Based Medicine,
 Oxford, UK 108
change
 barriers 104, 115, 119, 120–2
 emotional cycle 123–4
 implementation 125–6, 130
 management 118–19, 122–3, 127–31
 models 130–2
 monitoring and evaluation questions
  126–7
 planning 125

resistance to 122–3, 124–5
strategy development tools 127–31
checklists 88–9, 102, 113, 175, 177–82
    see also forms; questions
citation management 68
clinical decision support system (CDSS)
    128
clinical decision-making *see*
    decision-making
clinicians 30
Cochrane Collaboration 5–6, 96, 175
Cochrane Database of Systematic Reviews
    54, 65
cohort studies 78–9, 181
communication 126, 148, 165–6
confounding factors identification 80
congruity 81–2
consensus vs. evidence 105
consumers
    decision-making involvement 139
    evidence 30–1, 34–5
    guideline development involvement
        112–13
    information requirements 34
    participation 163–4
    roles 10–11
    systematic reviews 23
    see also patients
cost effectiveness 6, 84–6, 158, 161
creative adoption 133
criteria
    checklist, research paper weaknesses
        88–9
    critical appraisal 77–8
    exclusion 92, 102
    inclusion 59–60, 83, 92, 102, 174
    outcome 144
    process 144, 145
    qualitative data synthesis 95
    quality assessment 61–2
    quantitative 143–4
    structure 144–5, 147
    validity 80, 81, 83
critical appraisal *see* appraisal, critical
criticisms 11–14
culture 45, 92, 131
Cumulative Index to Nursing & Allied
    Health (CINAHL) database 65
Current Contents index 65

data
    analysis 43, 92–5
    collection
        issues 134
        methods 43, 82, 91

questions 54, 63–4, 126–7, 174
tools 62, 89–92, 145, 175–6, 183–6
    see also literature, searching
continuous 94, 184
dichotomous 93, 184
evaluation 145
presentation 94–5
sources 145
synthesis 62, 95–6, 176
    see also evidence; knowledge
Database of Abstracts of Reviews of
    Effects (DARE) 54, 65–6
database searching 54, 65–9, 115–16,
    174–5
    see also information technology
decision-making
    decision support system (DSS) 128–9
    evidence-based 4–5, 17
    information sources 31
    knowledge requirements 28
    resource allocation 156–7
    toolkits
        change evaluation 149
        change implementation 130
        clinical guidelines development 105
        evidence translation 30
        research evidence quality 89
        research evidence types 49
        search strategy 64
demands 3
developing countries, health care
    development 7–8
diagnosis 63
diagnostic analysis 138–9
dialectic transaction 41–2
diffusion of innovation model 129, 131–2
dissemination 107, 144
dissertation abstracts 66–7
dissonance 125
dropout 78, 79, 80
DSS (decision support system) 128–9

education 127–8, 139, 147, 162
effectiveness
    assessment tool 151
    cost- 6, 158
    defined 20–1, 28, 29–30, 139
    evidence sources 50
    improvement 8, 138
    increase desire 6
    interventions 4–5, 92
    model 18, 20, 36, 96–7, 111, 154
    outcomes 8, 140
    randomised controlled trials (RCTs)
        30

reviews 93
  strategies implementation 151
Einstein, Albert 16, 36
Embase database 66
ethical issues 134
ethnography 45, 49
evaluation 83–6, 133–5
  see also audit, clinical
evidence
  applicability levels 108, 109, 112
  generation 18–21, 36–51
  hierarchy tables 108, 110
  legal definition 31–2
  qualitative 81–3
  quality 88, 89, 107–8
  transfer into practice 119–20, 125–6,
    130–1, 149–50
  types 49
  utilisation 25, 118–36, 137–52
  see also data; findings; knowledge
evidence-based medicine (EBM) defined
    1, 5
evidence-based practice centres
  Australasian Cochrane Centre 7
  Australian Centre for Evidence-based
    Clinical Practice 150
  Centre for Evidence-Based Medicine,
    Oxford, UK 108, 109
  establishment 6–7, 10
  National Health Service (NHS) Centre
    for Reviews and Dissemination
    (NHS CRD) 7, 137, 138, 175
  see also Joanna Briggs Institute (JBI)
exclusion criteria 92, 102
experience 33
experts 23, 32, 33, 86–8, 134

FAME (Feasibility Appropriateness
    Meaningfulness Effectiveness)
    model 18, 20, 36, 96–7, 111, 154
feasibility
  defined 19, 28
  evidence sources 19, 28, 49
  interventions 92
  model 18, 20, 36, 96–7, 111, 154
  practice implementation 64, 73
Feasibility Appropriateness
    Meaningfulness Effectiveness
    (FAME) model 18, 20, 36, 96–7,
    111, 154
feedback process 129, 130, 138, 147
feminist research 48–9
findings 22, 64–9, 95, 149
  see also data; evidence
fixed effect model 94

forms 56, 90, 177–86
  see also checklists; information, sheets
Foucalt's definition of discourse 87
funding bodies, clinical audit
    involvement 141

Getting Research Into Practice (GRIP) 151
GIN (Guidelines International Network)
    103, 115
goals, clinical audit 140
government, clinical audit involvement
    141
graphs 94–5, 102
GRIP (Getting Research Into Practice) 151
guidelines
  allied-health-specific 104
  appraisal presentation 114
  basis 101
  clinical defined 103
  critical appraisal checklists and tools
    113–14, 177–82
  development
    consumer involvement 112–13
    defining best practice 143
    evidence use promotion 9
    sources 149
    strategies 6, 100–1, 105–7
    tools 115–16
  establishment framework 140
  implementation 118–36
  improved compliance 165
  medicine-specific 104
  nursing-specific 104
  paradigms 38–42
  revision requirement 107
  role 114–15, 161
  see also care standards
Guidelines International Network (GIN)
    103, 115

Habarmas, Jurgen 46–7
health, improvement, global 17, 19
hermeneutics 47
High Technology Assessment Database
    66

inclusion criteria 59–60, 83, 92, 102, 174
indicators 143–4
information
  access 148
  collection 91
  decision-making sources 31
  management 96–7, 157, 175, 176
  requirements, consumers 34
  sheets 102, 113, 175, 177–82

systems 128
see also data; evidence; knowledge
information technology 164–6
see also database searching
initiatives 10, 101, 152
innovation 129, 131–2
interests, human 46–7
International Guideline Library 115
internet 67
interventions
cost-benefit analysis 84
defined 90, 91
evaluation 92
identification 37
smoking cessation 27, 87, 100, 173–6
types 174

Joanna Briggs Institute (JBI)
effectiveness improvement role 8
establishment, Australia 7
evidence hierarchy adoption 108, 110
guidelines development 103
model 18, 27, 96–7, 154, 166–7
nursing practice evidence need 17
online libraries 115–16
outcomes effectiveness improvement
8
review protocol 55, 56
journal searching 68
see also database searching; literature,
searching

King, Witney, Jnr. 118
knowledge
generation 39
interests 46–7
management 156
practical defined 46
requirements, decision-making 28
transfer 24
translation 133
see also data; evidence; experts;
opinion
knowledge and human interests 46
knowledge retention from postoperative
patient information 58, 59–60

legal definition of evidence 31–2
legal implications 158, 159–61
legal regulation 156
librarian help 67, 68–9
Lincoln, Abraham 154
literature
data synthesis 62
evaluation 57

quality 102
reviews 6, 22, 101
searching 65, 67–70
see also database searching
selection 59, 60

managers 141, 156–7
marketing 127, 130
mean difference 94
meaningfulness
critical appraisal purpose 89
data 93
defined 20, 28, 29
evidence sources 50
evidence types 49
model 18, 20, 36, 96–7, 111, 154
understanding the experience 64
within defined cultural or geographical
context 73
Medline database 66
mental health 10
meta-analysis 12, 21–2, 93, 94
see also quantitative methods
meta-synthesis 23, 95
see also qualitative methods
methodology
approaches 31, 81–2
clinical audit 149
data collection 43, 82, 91
meta-analysis 12, 21–2, 93, 94
meta-synthesis 23, 95
phenomenology 45
research 31, 43, 47, 81–2
reviews 23, 32, 52, 54–5
statistical analysis 22–3, 78
study method appropriateness 78–9
see also qualitative methods;
quantitative methods
models
behaviour, social influence 129
for change 130–2
construction 166–7
evidence for practice 27–35
FAME 18, 20, 36, 96–7, 111, 154
fixed effect 94
mathematical 94
PACES 150–1
PDSA 131
random effects 94
reviews 96–7, 175, 176
SUMARI 96–7, 175, 176
transtheoretical 132
Monash Institute of Health Services
Research 7
mud map, research approaches 37–8

National Guidelines Clearing House 115
National Health and Medical Research
    Council (NHMRC) 116, 120
National Health Service (NHS) 163–4
National Health Service (NHS) Centre for
    Reviews and Dissemination (NHS
    CRD) 7, 137, 138, 175
National Institute for Clinical Studies 152
National Institute for Health and Clinical
    Excellence (NICE) 103, 152
National Institutes of Health 6, 100
negligence 160–2
NHMRC (National Health and Medical
    Research Council) 116, 120
nurses, clinical audit involvement 140–1

objectives 149
odds ratio 93
opinion 23, 32, 75, 86–8, 129
optimism 123
organisational context 156–7
organisations 103, 104
orientation, cultural and theoretical,
    researchers 82
outcomes
    assessment criteria 80
    continuous data 94, 184
    cost-benefit analysis 84
    criteria 144, 145
    effectiveness improvement 8
    improvement 3, 165
    measure
        blinding 78, 79
        cost 85
        form 184
        quality life years (QALY) 84
        reporting 90
        types 174
Oxford Centre for Evidence-Based
    Medicine, evidence levels 109

PACES (Practical Application of Clinical
    Evidence System) 150–1
paradigm 38–42, 43, 46, 47
participant representation 83
participant types 174
patients
    clinical effectiveness focus 140
    demands 3
    follow-up 78, 79
    hospitalised, smoking cessation
        strategies 173–6
    involvement 148
    see also consumers; smoking cessation
PDSA (plan-do-study-act) model 131

Pearson, A.
    alternative approaches 30–1
    document text examination processes
        86–7
    evidence evaluation 111
    pluralistic approach 32, 34–5
    qualitative data synthesis 95
    validity criteria 81–3
pessimism 123
phenomenology 44–5, 50
philosophers 31–2, 39, 46
philosophy 44–5, 81
plan-do-study-act (PDSA) model 131
planning
    action plan 146–7
    change 125
    clinical audit 141–2, 146
    practice improvement 149
    urban 162–3
policy 158, 162–3
positivism 38–41, 43, 46
Practical Application of Clinical Evidence
    System (PACES) 150–1
practice
    best 6, 9, 142–3, 144
    development 3
    grounded in theory 13, 16
    identification 37
    implementation feasibility 64, 73
    improvement, planned 149
    information sheets 102, 113, 175, 177–82
    recommendations 105, 106, 107–12
    theory, embedded in 41
praxis 47
presentation 94–5, 106–7, 114
prevention 64
process criteria 144, 145
professionals, health 3–4, 32–3, 140–1
prognosis 63
programme evaluation 134
proposal development 54
PsycINFO database 65

qualitative methods
    best available evidence base 30–1
    consumer information research 34
    data extraction 90–2
    data synthesis criteria 95–6
    qualitative/quantitative debate 40,
        42–3
    research evidence assessment,
        standards 81
    research review methods, evolving 32
    results synthesis 23
    systematic reviews inclusion 35

quality
  analysis 138–9
  assessment, research 61–2, 103, 115–16
  assurance 134
  care 113, 139, 159
  continuous monitoring and
      improvement 165
  quality life years (QALY) 84
  reporting 80, 83
  studies 89
  see also audit, clinical; care standards
quantitative methods
  criteria 143–4
  data extraction 89–90
  positivist paradigm 39–40
  quantitative/qualitative debate 40,
      42–3
  results synthesis 22
  systematic review example 54–5
  systematic reviews inclusion 35
  see also randomised controlled trials
      (RCTs)
quasi-experimental studies 44, 77–8
questions 63–4, 126–7, 174
  see also checklists

random effects model 94
randomised controlled trials (RCTs)
  critical appraisal 76, 77–8
  effectiveness 4, 30
  evidence-based practice reliance on 12
  guidelines development basis 105
  limitation 16–17, 32, 35
  systematic review 5–6
  validity 75–6
  see also quantitative methods
rationalism, economic 161
re-auditing 147
realism, hopeful 123
reality defined 44–5
recommendations, grading 105, 106,
      107–12
references 102
reminders 128, 130
report writing 100, 102, 148–9
reporting quality 80, 83
research
  approaches 37–8, 44–9
  defined 37
  experimental 43–4
  feminist 48–9
  paper weaknesses checklist 88–9
  process rigour 74–5, 86, 113–14
  quality assessment 61–2
  quasi-experimental 44

review methods 32
  theoretical underpinnings 91
  utilisation 157
  weighed with internal sources 34
  see also methodology; qualitative
      methods; quantitative methods;
      randomised controlled trials
      (RCTs); systematic reviews
research and development (R&D)
      strategies development 6–7, 101
researchers orientations 82–3
resistance to change 122–3, 124–5
resource allocation, decision-making
      156–7
Review Manager (RevMan) 96, 176
reviews *see* systematic reviews
reviews, systematic
  administrators other disciplines 134
  critical appraisal 74–5
  databases 54, 65–6
  defined 101
  effectiveness 93
  guidelines 101, 104
  literature 6, 22, 101
  management 96, 176
  methods 23, 32, 52, 54–5
  models 96–7, 175, 176
  objectives 58, 102
  peer 149
  protocol 52, 54, 55–63, 102, 173–6
  questions 54, 174
  reports 100, 101, 102
  study selection 69–70
  synthesis 21, 52–71
  theory 52
  title 56
  see also randomised controlled trials
      (RCTs)
RevMan (Review Manager) 96, 176
rigour 74–5, 86, 113–14
risk 93–4
Russell, Bertrand 27

Schutz, Alfred 41
Schweitzer, Albert 99
Science Citation Index 66
Scottish Intercollegiate Guidelines
      Network (SIGN) 103, 115
search strategy 60–1, 174–5
self-consciousness 47
self-improvement 64
self-knowledge 46–7
sensitivity analysis 85–6
SIGN (Scottish Intercollegiate Guidelines
      Network) 103, 115

Silagy, Chris 7
situation analysis 126–7
smoking cessation
    acupuncture effectiveness 37, 41, 51, 54
    advice provision establishment 146–7
    appropriate review question 54, 55
    cultural influence 53, 79
    evidence requirements 33, 35
    feasibility evidence 28
    guidelines 138
    interventions and strategies 27, 87, 100, 173–6
    knowledge translation 133
    literature identification 73
    quantitative review 54–5
    randomised controlled trials (RCTs) 77
    review protocol development 57
    unsuccessful 2, 4
social influence model of behaviour 129
sources
    alternative to research 33–4
    clinical questions 63–4
    data 145
    decision-making information 31
    effectiveness evidence 50
    evidence generation link 20–1
    guidelines development 149
    identification 87
    meaningfulness 50
    valid forms 23
stakeholders 113, 140–1
    see also consumers
standardised differences in mean 94
standards 23, 81
    see also care standards
statistical analysis 22–3, 78
    see also meta-analysis
strategies
    audit 148
    change management 127–31
    development, research and development (R&D) 6–7, 101
    guidelines development 6, 100–1, 105–7
    implementation effectiveness 151
    search 60–1, 64–5, 174
    smoking cessation 27, 87, 100, 173–6
structure criteria 144–5, 147
studies
    description 102
    interpretive 81–3
    method appropriateness 78
    results form 184
    selection 52, 69–70
    types 174

SUMARI (System for Unified Management of the Assessment and Review of Information) 96–7, 175, 176
symbolic interactionist theory 45
synthesis
    data 62, 95–6, 176
    defined 96
    economic analysis 23
    evaluations 23
    explained 21–4
    findings 22
    systematic review 21, 52–71
    see also meta-synthesis
system changing 147
System for Unified Management of the Assessment and Review of Information (SUMARI) 96–7, 175, 176

teamwork 148
textual pooling 176
theoretical premises 81
theory
    action 42
    critical 46, 47
    diffusion theory of innovation 129
    embedded in practice 41
    evidence synthesis element 21
    grounded 16, 45, 49
    practice gap 133
    practice grounded in 13
    quantitative 39
    symbolic interactionist 45
    systematic review element 52
therapy 64
thesauri 67
three-point level, evidence scale 108
time, dedicated 148
time frame 134
tools
    audit 149–51
    change strategy development 127–31
    checklists 88–9, 102, 113, 175, 177–82
    data collection/extraction 62, 89–92, 145, 175–6, 183–6
    effectiveness assessment 151
    guideline development 113–14, 115–16
    systematic review 53, 96–7
    see also audit, clinical; decision-making, toolkits; models
topic choosing 142–3
tradition, health care role 33
training 148

transfer, evidence into practice 24,
        119–20, 125–6, 130–1, 149–50
transtheoretical model 132
truncation 67

validity
  assessment 86
  cohort studies 181
  criteria 80, 81, 83, 88

defined 74–5
establishment 87
FAME model 111

weighted mean difference 94
wild card 67
world wide web 67
writing 47, 102, 148–9